ARTHRITIS-PROOF YOUR LIFE

ARTHRITIS-PROOF YOUR LIFE

SECRETS TO PAIN-FREE LIVING WITHOUT DRUGS

MICHELLE SCHOFFRO COOK, PhD, DNC, ROHP

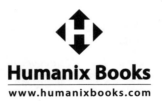

Humanix Books

www.humanixbooks.com

Humanix Books

Arthritis-Proof Your Life
Copyright © 2016 by Humanix Books
All rights reserved

Humanix Books, P.O. Box 20989, West Palm Beach, FL 33416, USA
www.humanixbooks.com | info@humanixbooks.com

Library of Congress Cataloging-in-Publication Data

Names: Cook, Michelle Schoffro, author.
Title: Arthritis-proof your life : secrets to pain-free living without drugs /
Michelle Schoffro Cook.
Description: West Palm Beach, FL : Humanix Books, 2016. | Includes index.
Identifiers: LCCN 2016010738 (print) | LCCN 2016022999 (ebook) | ISBN
9781630060626 (hardback) | ISBN 9781630060633 (eBook)
Subjects: LCSH: Arthritis—Alternative treatment—Popular works. | Arthritis—
Diet therapy—Popular works. | Arthritis—Diet therapy—Recipes. | BISAC:
HEALTH & FITNESS / Diseases / Immune System. | HEALTH & FITNESS /
Alternative Therapies. | HEALTH & FITNESS / Pain Management. | HEALTH
& FITNESS / Naturopathy.
Classification: LCC RC933 .C679 2016 (print) | LCC RC933 (ebook) | DDC
616.7/220654—dc23
LC record available at https://lccn.loc.gov/2016010738

Cover Photo: Visions of America, LLC / Alamy, EHMPJD
Cover Design: Tom Lau
Interior Design: Scribe, Inc.

Humanix Books is a division of Humanix Publishing, LLC. Its trademark, con-
sisting of the words "Humanix" is registered in the Patent and Trademark Office
and in other countries.

Disclaimer: The information presented in this book is meant to be used for
general resource purposes only; it is not intended as specific medical advice
for any individual and should not substitute medical advice from a healthcare
professional. If you have (or think you may have) a medical problem, speak to
your doctor or healthcare practitioner immediately about your risk and possible
treatments. Do not engage in any therapy or treatment without consulting a
medical professional.

ISBN: 978-1-63006-062-6 (Hardcover)
ISBN: 978-1-63006-063-3 (E-book)

Printed in the United States of America
10 9 8 7 6 5 4 3

Dedication

I dedicate this book to my parents, Michael and Deborah Schoffro. Thank you for always believing in me and my writing and for being wonderful parents and great friends.

I also dedicate this book to Dr. Robert Laquerre at Alta Vista Chiropractic, in Ottawa, Ontario, Canada. Your caring and compassionate approach to health care transformed my quality of life many years ago and helped me to live the life I dreamed about.

Acknowledgments

TO THE MANY WONDERFUL people who helped make this book happen, including:

Curtis Cook, the love of my life, my husband, and my soul mate. I am eternally grateful for your love and am so thrilled to spend my life with you. Thank you for your constant care, love, friendship, and support. There is no better man than you.

Claire Gerus, thank you. You are a visionary agent and a great friend. I appreciate your ongoing efforts to secure my books and your many insights throughout my career.

Mary Glenn, thanks for your support of my work and vision for this book. I appreciate it.

Michael and Deborah Schoffro, thank you, Mom and Dad. You have always been so supportive of my writing and have been wonderful parents. Thank you for your encouragement and love.

To the team at Humanix, thanks for your many efforts to bring this book to those people suffering from arthritis and fibromyalgia.

Table of Contents

INTRODUCTION

What Your Doctor Isn't Telling You *Is* Hurting You!

ANYONE WHO HAS EXPERIENCED the debilitating pain and inflammation of arthritis will tell you how much these symptoms can rob you of the joy of living, from the pleasure of pursuing a beloved hobby to the satisfaction of enjoying a favorite sport. For some people arthritis pain can interfere with their ability to perform even the simplest tasks and often prevents sufferers from getting that much needed, restorative good night's sleep.

According to the Centers for Disease Control and Prevention (CDC), an estimated 50 million adults in the United States have been diagnosed as having rheumatoid arthritis, gout, lupus, or fibromyalgia. Although many of these people are mature adults, this debilitating disease affects even children. The CDC estimates that 294,000 children under eighteen have been diagnosed with some form of arthritic or rheumatic condition.

It is now estimated that almost half of Americans will receive an osteoarthritis (OA) diagnosis in their lifetime. And for the millions of people who are overweight, two out of three are likely to develop osteoarthritis.

Although drugs may temporarily relieve some of the pain, the flip side is potentially serious: the list of side effects can be worse than the disease itself, particularly when it comes to drugs that have been linked to many deaths. Sadly many of these drugs continue to be marketed as the only options for people suffering from arthritis, which is patently untrue.

What is *arthritis*? The diagnosis simply means inflammation of the joints. But it doesn't tell you what caused the joint inflammation. Although drugs may reduce the pain in some people, they don't address the underlying causes or underlying issues in the body that can lead to arthritis. That's exactly what this book will address—the root causes of arthritis. More importantly, *Arthritis-Proof Your Life: The Drug-Free, All-Natural Way to Beat Pain and Inflammation* offers you an opportunity to discover your body's potential underlying weaknesses such as nutritional deficiencies, bodily imbalances, and lifestyle choices so you can get to the bottom of what's causing the inflammation in your body—and get rid of it! Addressing the root causes of arthritis is much more effective than taking a drug-based Band-Aid approach that merely lessens symptoms.

When it comes to arthritis, what your doctor doesn't know *is* hurting you. *Arthritis-Proof Your Life* works by resetting your natural body chemistry and addressing the underlying causal factors for arthritis instead of undergoing the medical approach, which reduces symptoms at a high cost to the body. As you will soon discover, cutting-edge research shows that low-grade inflammation, nutritional deficiencies, food sensitivities, infections, and an inflammatory diet puts you at risk of experiencing arthritis or aggravating the pain and inflammation of arthritis.

But it's not enough to know the factors causing or aggravating your symptoms; you need to know how to effectively overcome these issues to reduce your pain, heal your joints, and live the life you deserve to live.

In *Arthritis-Proof Your Life* I will reveal how you can eat to beat inflammation, identify food sensitivities, reverse nutritional deficiencies, and heal the infections and imbalances linked to arthritis. You will learn how to restore proper pain signals to your brain and decrease inflammation in your joints. This book will even reveal exciting, advanced research that shows the key to pain relief is to speed up your body's natural inflammatory response so it can "clean up" the joints and dramatically reduce pain. That's probably not something your doctor has ever told you.

You'll find dozens of scientifically proven natural therapies and remedies for arthritis that have never before been compiled into a single book and many of which are virtually unknown—the product of my twenty-five years of research and experience in the natural health field. I am a registered nutritionist, board-certified doctor of natural medicine, certified herbalist, doctor of acupuncture, and the author of eighteen other natural health books. I spend almost every day researching the best proven natural medicines to help people overcome illnesses they may believe are incurable. My quest to offer the best healing advice for treating arthritis and pain disorders has led me to research new and advanced natural treatments, including potent phytonutrients that combat joint damage, enzyme therapy to alleviate both pain and inflammation, and orthomolecular therapy that halts the progression of the disease. My clients and readers alike regularly share their successes in transforming their health and improving their quality of life.

I compiled this information into one book in my quest to empower you, the reader, to take charge of your life and to put health and healing information into a practical, do-it-yourself format that is easy to follow and use. I hope you will experience a health transformation.

In chapter 1 you'll learn more about the medical view of arthritis as compared to a holistic one and explore some of the dangers of common arthritis medications. In chapter 2 you'll discover the most common foods that cause or worsen inflammation in your body and aggravate arthritis as well as the healing anti-inflammatory foods and spices you can add to your diet to help boost your body's innate healing capacity. In chapter 3 you'll uncover a little-known nutritional cause of arthritis and how correcting it can have a huge impact on slowing the disease's progression and may halt the disease in its tracks. In chapter 4 you'll discover the miracle warriors that fight against arthritis to reduce swelling and inflammation and speed the healing process. In chapter 5 you'll learn about natural medicines that work against arthritis, everything from probiotics to herbs. Chapter 6 will help you put pain reduction at your fingertips in the form of acupressure. If you think aromatherapy is just about baths and spa treatments, you'll be pleasantly surprised to learn in chapter 7 that a form of medical aromatherapy is showing huge promise against the symptoms of arthritis and may even help restore normal pain signals in the brain, which in turn reduces pain levels. In chapter 8 you'll learn about other therapies and natural approaches to arthritis that will improve your quality of life. And finally, in chapter 9 you'll enjoy delicious and nutritious healing recipes that can help you integrate arthritis-healing foods into your day-to-day life. It includes recipes like Dr. Cook's Ginger Pain-Relief Tea, Celery-Apple Anti-Inflammatory Juice, Happy Joint Juice, Anti-Arthritis Powerhouse Salad, and Ultimate Joint-Healing Curry.

Unlike many books that offer plenty of theory but few practical solutions, *Arthritis-Proof Your Life* offers you a wide variety of both cutting-edge and tried-and-true natural therapies without the harmful side effects of common arthritis drugs. Whether you're coping with the debilitating effects of rheumatoid arthritis, osteoarthritis, gout, fibromyalgia, or another form of arthritis, *Arthritis-Proof Your Life* gives you all the tools you'll need to enjoy pain-free living and an improved quality of life.

1

A Medical and Holistic View of Arthritis

BARBARA, AN ELEGANT, WELL-DRESSED, and seemingly wealthy woman in her fifties, came to see me for rheumatoid arthritis. She had suffered from the condition for many years and had been taking the pharmaceutical drug Celebrex for just over a year when she arrived in my office. Frequent media reports of several deaths linked to the drug had caught her attention, and she was concerned that the drug might not be as safe as her doctor and pharmacist had told her.

As with all of my patients, I went through an exhaustive medical and personal history with Barbara. In my twenty-five years of experience as a clinical nutritionist, doctor of natural medicine, and doctor of acupuncture, I have found that seemingly unrelated aspects of a person's life are often linked to the condition they are suffering from, so it was important I discover anything that might be playing a role in Barbara's health. Whereas the drug-based approach is only concerned with symptoms, I have found that a person is far more than a collection of symptoms, so doling out the same drugs for different patients is rarely an effective long-term strategy.

Barbara and I discussed her joint pain that she largely found in her knees, her use of the drug Celebrex, and her marriage, which she indicated was strong. Because her arthritis symptoms began about a year after her move into her current field of work, we proceeded to explore her professional life to identify any possible stresses that may be triggering a cascade of stress hormones and the resulting aggravation of inflammation in her body. Barbara said she and her husband had owned a large ranch when they both worked in the oil and gas industry, and she also worked as a management consultant assisting many companies in various temporary roles on an as-needed basis.

When I asked her whether she enjoyed her work she indicated that "it was a job"; she clearly derived no pleasure from it at all. She said it was difficult, and although she enjoyed the intellectual challenge, she hated the extremely sexist environment. She explained that she had been "hit on" by many of her male colleagues at multiple corporations and shared that these men routinely made lewd comments about women, shared misogynistic jokes, and generally treated women as nothing more than sex objects. Because she found it increasingly difficult to get out of bed in the morning and recoiled at the thought of going to work each day, she had reduced her workload to part-time hours, working three days weekly. I asked Barbara whether she would consider switching to a different industry, as her managerial skills would obviously apply to other fields of work. She said she could but was concerned that it "would be too difficult" at her age and that, more importantly, she needed the extended healthcare benefits to pay for the Celebrex and other arthritis drugs, which cost her over a thousand dollars monthly. She felt trapped in a vicious cycle of needing to stay employed in a field of work that was harmful to her health just so she could pay for the drugs she needed to manage her symptoms.

Obviously her work was creating severe stress for Barbara, but we agreed to focus on building her health through natural means first so she could eventually get off of the drugs; doing so might enable her to pursue a different line of work if she no longer needed the medical insurance from the oil and gas corporations to pay for the pharmaceutical drugs. Barbara followed fairly closely the low-sugar, low-refined carbohydrate diet I recommended. We added to her program a supplement containing glucosamine sulfate, chondroitin, and MSM. I recommended a blend of vitamin D, selenium, and zinc along with an extract of the herb hops specifically formulated for autoimmune disorders like rheumatoid arthritis. I also prescribed the herb *Harpagophytum procumbens* (colloquially known as devil's claw), as I had found it was effective for easing joint pain and arthritis. She agreed to get fresh air and gentle walks daily but to rest when her joints severely ached. I also prescribed a high-potency multiprobiotic formula along with aloe vera juice to help heal Barbara's gut because I suspected it was playing a key role in the disease's progression.

Because she was eager to discontinue her medications, we agreed she should be monitored closely. As a result, she came back to see me every two weeks for the first two months and then monthly afterward. Within six months Barbara no longer needed Celebrex and could manage her arthritis entirely with the natural medicines I prescribed, which she took faithfully. She reported feeling significantly improved, relieved that she no longer needed or used Celebrex, and felt empowered from taking such control of her life.

After a few additional months Barbara announced she was making a career change. She said she realized that working in an environment that was so hostile to women was causing severe stress. Barbara asked me whether I thought pharmaceutical drugs could numb the emotions in addition to numbing pain. I indicated that I believed that some drugs could have this effect. She felt that the potent drugs she had been taking had prevented her from fully feeling the anger, outrage, and sadness she experienced from being exposed to such a misogynistic work environment.

Barbara was so amazed that the natural options had been such powerful healers that she decided to go back to school to train in a specialized form of healing within the natural health field. Barbara now travels worldwide with her husband lecturing on natural health topics and has her own online radio program and health consulting practice. She now feels a lot less stress, and is able to help others suffering from arthritis. Although she still has the condition, she experiences a significant reduction in arthritis pain because she is able to manage it using diet, lifestyle, and natural medicine.

WHAT EXACTLY IS ARTHRITIS?

You probably already have some insights into arthritis, but let's explore the disease briefly. Arthritis is a rheumatic condition that causes pain and inflammation in the joints. Rheumatic diseases and conditions affect the musculoskeletal system and can include abnormalities of the immune system. The term *arthritis* has become so common that we often forget how serious it can be.

Although there are numerous forms of arthritis, two of the two most common forms are osteoarthritis, which is a joint disease, and rheumatoid arthritis, which damages the connective tissue in our body and is considered an autoimmune disease. Autoimmune diseases involve the body's immune system mistakenly attacking healthy tissue, which can include the joints but tends to be throughout the body. Additionally, other conditions like fibromyalgia, gout, lupus, and scleroderma are also classified as types of arthritis.

Osteoarthritis

By far the most common form of arthritis, osteoarthritis takes hold when cartilage—a fibrous, elastic connective tissue found in joints and other parts of the body—begins to deteriorate and wear down. There are many reasons why this can happen, but two of the most common are injuries and excessive body weight, which puts additional pressure on the joints and the ligaments that hold them in place.

Rheumatoid Arthritis

Rheumatoid arthritis is a painful condition of the joints, but it is actually a body-wide condition. It most commonly affects the hands but frequently occurs in multiple places at once and can even affect the whole body, including fingers, elbows, wrists, and knees. Whereas it often starts in middle age, many younger people experience rheumatoid arthritis too. Although the symptoms are primarily *felt* in the joints, rheumatoid arthritis affects tissue connecting bones and joints in many places in the body. Nutritional deficiencies and even pathogens, such as bacterial, yeast, and fungal infections, can cause or worsen rheumatoid arthritis.

Fibromyalgia

Fibromyalgia is a type of arthritis. Doctors classify fibromyalgia as a syndrome, which means that it is a collection of seemingly unconnected symptoms, with the main one being unaccountable pain in the muscles (*myo* means muscle; *algia* means pain). The cause of syndromes is uncertain, but in the case of fibromyalgia, it often starts after an illness, injury, or trauma. In addition to pain, there are many other symptoms. The following are the diagnostic criteria for fibromyalgia:

- widespread pain in all four quadrants of the body lasting for at least three months

- tenderness in at least eleven of the eighteen specified tender points implicated in fibromyalgia
- generalized aches or stiffness of at least three anatomic sites for at least three months
- exclusion of other disorders that are known to cause similar symptoms

Additionally, there are other minor diagnostic criteria for fibromyalgia, which include:

- chronic headache
- sleep disturbance
- neurological and psychological complaints
- joint swelling
- numbing or tingling sensations
- irritable bowel syndrome
- variations of symptoms in relation to activity, stress, and weather changes
- temporomandibular joint syndrome (TMJ)

Gout

Gout is a painful form of arthritis that is usually linked to pain in the big toe. It occurs when uric acid in the blood causes crystals to form and accumulate around joints, particularly in the big toe.

So how does uric acid build up in the blood? There are many foods that, when metabolized, cause acidic buildup, especially meat, alcohol, and seafood. For more information about the specific foods that cause uric acid buildup, see page 65.

A JOINT PARTNERSHIP

Because having healthy joints is imperative to preventing or addressing arthritis, let's explore the components of the joints so we're better able to care for them. There are four main components of a joint: ligaments, cartilage, joint capsule, and bursae.

Ligaments

Ligaments are like straps that hold bones together at the joints to add stability. They can become damaged if a force acts too strongly against a joint. For example, ligaments stabilize the joints when bending sideways, but if a force pushes the joint too hard in that direction, the ligaments can become damaged. If ligaments are damaged, there is usually pain and swelling around the joint. Overstretching the ligaments can cause the joints to become unstable and affect their alignment and stability. Chronically weakened ligaments can occur anywhere, but they are especially prevalent around the shoulders, knees, and elbows.

Cartilage

The ends of bones are covered in cartilage to provide a smooth surface that absorbs some shock. However, damage to the cartilage can make the joints more susceptible to wear. Joints like the knees have additional cartilage to act like washers, filling in gaps between the bones that otherwise do not fit together perfectly.

Joint Capsules

The joint capsule is a type of ligament that forms a bag around the joint to contain a lubricating fluid known as synovial fluid. These capsules keep joints lubricated but can be injured in the same way as other ligaments.

Bursae

These fluid-filled sacs are positioned at key points around certain joints to act as cushions, separating and padding neighboring tissues. High amounts of overuse and stress on a joint can cause the bursa to become inflamed, resulting in swelling; for example, lengthy amounts of time kneeling can cause the bursa at the front of the knee to become sore and swollen. Although this damage frequently occurs in the knees, it can occur in any joint.

MEDICATIONS: HIGH RISK, LOW REWARD

When you consider the intense nature of pain and inflammation linked to arthritis, it may be hard to believe that the best remedies are the common foods found in your refrigerator or natural remedies available in many herbal dispensaries and health food stores. It may be far more tempting to believe the advertising we see on television, in magazines, and online for what we have been told are powerful prescription drugs to eliminate the pain. I urge you to question the drug myth that we have accepted in our society, the one that says drugs are the only—and even preferred option—for treating illnesses like arthritis.

Once a doctor gives you a diagnosis of arthritis, fibromyalgia, gout, or another type or arthritis-related condition, he or she proceeds to pull out the prescription pad for one or more drugs. Few doctors ever take the time or, perhaps more accurately, make the effort to get to the bottom of your symptoms. This may leave you thinking that the cause of arthritis is arthritis itself and never give its origins further consideration. Most people blame bad genes or, in the case of osteoarthritis, an old injury. And although genes and injuries can play a role in the condition, they are not the only factors. Before we delve into the many factors implicated in arthritis, let's first explore the likely prescriptions your doctor sent you home with and, indeed, you may already be taking.

Over the past few years the media has reported on the health controversies—and related lawsuits—of numerous pharmaceutical drugs for arthritis and inflammation. The debate around the safety and efficacy of arthritis medications like Celebrex has left many arthritis sufferers looking for safe, natural, and effective alternatives to prescription drugs. Fortunately nature provides an abundance of safe, powerful remedies in the form of herbs, foods, and nutritional supplements. But don't believe the prevailing mindset that natural options are not as powerful as drug options—that is merely a myth, as you'll discover later in this book. But first, let's explore some of the problems with the pharmaceutical drugs you may be taking to alleviate your arthritis symptoms.

Doctors write prescriptions for pain medications because people want fast and simple pain relief (or some other type of relief) without wanting to make changes to their lives, namely changing eating and lifestyle habits. As an aside, the vast majority of medical doctors have no training in healthy eating, so they cannot provide dietary advice to their patients. The only advice given in most medical consultation rooms involves how and when to take a particular prescription or two—or maybe even three or more drugs.

That's a scary thought. Drug interactions and side effects as well as overlooked contraindications remain a serious problem in North America and frequently lead to somber side effects and sometimes even death. Millions of people do not understand how to take their medications correctly or choose to ignore instructions, abuse prescriptions, or neglect to inform new doctors and pharmacists about the drugs they are taking, all of which can lead to misprescribing or duplicating prescriptions and overall healthcare error. And that's just the incorrect use of drugs.

The *correct* use of drugs is also a serious threat to health. Sadly, death by prescription drugs is a far more common problem than death from illicit drugs. More people die at the hand of the prescription pad than from taking illegal street drugs. Additionally, more people die from prescription drug use than from traffic accidents.[1]

Do Arthritis Drugs Scare You? They Should!

The side effects associated with pharmaceutical drugs have become a serious concern to arthritis sufferers. More and more people question whether the side effects of the drugs, which in some cases can include death, may be worse than the original condition. In a recent advertisement found in a popular women's magazine for the rheumatoid arthritis drug Cimzia (certolizumab pegol), one page was devoted to how the drug could help with rheumatoid arthritis. Once you flipped the page, however, two full pages showcased the "safety information" and the "consumer brief"—the serious side effects of taking the drug. The side effects of this drug included heart failure, cancer, multiple sclerosis, seizures, hepatitis B reactivation, breathing problems, blood problems, flu, colds, bladder infections, rash, and psoriasis. Based on this lengthy list of side effects, arthritis may be the least of your problems. And I am in no way intending to diminish the seriousness of arthritis here.

Common Medications for Arthritis

There are many common arthritis drugs. In a study published in the medical journal *Rheumatology News*, analyzing 7,945,910 prescriptions written by rheumatologists over three months, the six most commonly prescribed medications along with the percentage of arthritis sufferers that use them included:

1. methotrexate (8.5 percent)
2. prednisone (7.7 percent)
3. folic acid (5.8 percent)
4. hydroxychloroquine (5.7 percent)
5. hydrocodone and acetaminophen (4.5 percent)
6. tramadol (2.3 percent)[2]

Other common drugs for rheumatoid arthritis include (the percentage of prescriptions written for each drug follows in parentheses) meloxicam (2.1 percent), Celebrex (celecoxib) (1.9 percent), cyclobenzaprine (1.6 percent), and Lyrica (pregabalin) (1.6 percent).

Let's explore the five most commonly used arthritis drugs, excluding folic acid, which is actually a nutrient and will be discussed later in this book. We will investigate the many side effects and nutrient, herb, and food interactions of these drugs so you can better decide whether these pharmaceutical treatments are right for you if you're already taking them or plan to take them. Of course, you should always consult your physician if you are interested in discontinuing any medication, particularly ones you have been taking for more than a few months, as you may need to be slowly weaned off the prescription and undergo medical observation during this process.

METHOTREXATE

Methotrexate is a chemotherapy drug that is also used for arthritis. It can cause a long list of side effects, some of which include:[3]

- back pain
- black, tarry stools
- blood in the urine or stools
- bloody vomit
- blurred vision
- confusion
- convulsions (seizures)
- cough or hoarseness
- dark urine
- diarrhea
- dizziness
- drowsiness
- fever or chills
- headache
- joint pain
- lower back or side pain

- painful or difficult urination
- pinpoint red spots on the skin
- reddening of the skin
- shortness of breath
- sores in the mouth or lips
- stomach pain
- swelling of the feet or lower legs
- unusual bleeding or bruising
- unusual tiredness or weakness
- yellow eyes or skin

Because it blocks the activation of folic acid (vitamin B9) in the body, you may need supplementary folic acid along with methotrexate to lessen or alleviate side effects linked with the drug.[4] As you may have guessed from seeing folic acid on the list of most commonly prescribed arthritis drugs, the nutrient is a highly effective treatment for arthritis, so any drug that depletes this vitamin may actually aggravate arthritis, particularly over the long term. Vitamin B9 is imperative for sufficient cellular energy and healthy joints.

There are some beneficial natural supplements that help reduce the harmful effects of this drug, including beta carotene, chamomile, eleuthero (ginseng), folic acid, ginger, glutamine, spleen peptide extract, vitamin A, and zinc. The antioxidants glutamine, melatonin, milk thistle, and PSK may also be beneficial.[5] Follow package instructions for the specific products you choose. Avoid using PABA while taking methotrexate, as the combination may cause an adverse reaction.

PREDNISONE

Prednisone is a synthetic anti-inflammatory corticosteroid drug with a lengthy list of possible side effects, some of which include:[6]

- abdominal or stomach pain or burning sensations
- abnormal fat deposits on the face, neck, and trunk

- acne
- aggression
- agitation
- anxiety
- backache
- bloody, black, or tarry stools
- blurred vision
- cough or hoarseness
- decreased vision
- depression
- diarrhea
- dizziness
- dry mouth
- dry scalp
- eye pain or tearing
- facial hair growth in females
- fainting
- fast, slow, pounding, or irregular heartbeat or pulse
- fever or chills
- fractures
- full or round face, neck, or trunk
- headache
- heartburn or indigestion (severe and continuous)
- increased appetite and thirst
- irritability
- loss of sexual desire or ability
- lower back or side pain
- menstrual irregularities
- mood changes
- muscle pain or tenderness, or muscle weakness
- nausea
- nervousness
- numbness or tingling in the arms or legs
- pain in back, ribs, arms, or legs

- painful or difficult urination
- reddish purple lines on the arms, face, legs, trunk, or groin
- shortness of breath
- sleeplessness
- sweating
- swelling of the fingers, hands, feet, or lower legs
- thinning of the scalp hair
- unusual tiredness or weakness
- vision changes
- vomiting
- weight gain

Research has shown that ongoing prednisone use can cause the depletion of calcium, chromium, magnesium, melatonin (hormone), potassium, selenium, and vitamins B6 and D (hormone). Supplementation with these nutrients and melatonin may be beneficial.[7] Supplemental chromium and vitamin A may also reduce side effects. Additionally, N-acetyl cysteine (NAC) may increase the effectiveness of prednisone in the body, so you may need less of the medication.[8] Follow package directions for the specific nutritional and herbal products you choose.

Adverse reactions have been reported between prednisone and the use of alcohol or sodium. Use of diuretic herbs such as buckthorn or alder buckthorn should be undertaken with caution, as they can cause the loss of potassium. Corticosteroids like prednisone can also deplete this essential electrolyte nutrient. In test-tube studies, licorice extract caused the detoxification of prednisone, so you should not use this herb while taking prednisone without first consulting a physician. Other diuretic herbs that should be avoided include asparagus root, butcher's broom, cleavers, corn silk, juniper, maté, and parsley.[9] Follow package directions for the specific nutritional and herbal products you choose. People taking prednisone may have higher protein needs than the average person because this drug can cause a loss of protein. Grapefruit juice may increase the effects of corticosteroids and should, therefore, be avoided or used only under a physician's direction.

HYDROXYCHLOROQUINE

Hydroxychloroquine is classified as an antimalarial drug that is also used for treating rheumatoid arthritis. The following are some of the side effects of taking this drug:[10]

- bleaching of hair or increased hair loss
- blue-black discoloration of skin, fingernails, or inside of mouth
- blurred vision or any other change in vision
- convulsions (seizures)
- diarrhea
- difficulty in seeing to read
- dizziness or lightheadedness
- headache
- increased muscle weakness
- itching (more common in black patients)
- loss of appetite
- mood or other mental changes
- nausea or vomiting
- nervousness or restlessness
- ringing or buzzing in ears or any loss of hearing
- skin rash
- sore throat and fever
- stomach cramps or pain
- unusual bleeding or bruising
- unusual tiredness
- weakness

The drug may block the formation of vitamin D in the body and deplete calcium, so you may need to supplement with both nutrients while taking hydroxychloroquine. Excessive magnesium may reduce drug absorption and should, therefore, be avoided while taking this drug.[11] Follow package directions for the specific nutritional and herbal products you choose.

HYDROCODONE

Hydrocodone is a narcotic analgesic used with acetaminophen, a nonsteroidal anti-inflammatory drug (NSAID). Some of the side effects include:[12]

- abdominal or stomach pain or discomfort
- back pain
- bladder pain
- bloating or swelling of the face, arms, hands, lower legs, or feet
- bloody or cloudy urine
- body aches or pain
- chills
- cough
- depression
- difficult or labored breathing
- difficult, burning, or painful urination
- difficulty having a bowel movement (stool)
- dry mouth
- ear congestion
- fear or nervousness
- fever
- frequent urge to urinate
- headache
- heartburn
- itching skin
- loss of voice
- lower back or side pain
- muscle spasms

- nasal congestion
- nausea
- rapid weight gain
- runny nose
- sneezing
- sore throat
- tightness in the chest
- tingling of the hands or feet
- unusual tiredness or weakness
- unusual weight gain or loss
- vomiting

There are no known drug-nutrient-herb interactions for hydrocodone. Because the drug may cause gastrointestinal upset, taking it with food may help counter this side effect. Hydrocodone may also cause constipation, so a high-fiber diet and plenty of water may be beneficial. Avoid drinking alcohol, as it can intensify the drug's effects.

ACETAMINOPHEN

Best known as Tylenol, acetaminophen is a drug arthritis sufferers use to address pain. Although it may help reduce pain, it does not reduce the underlying inflammation of arthritis, causing acetaminophen to be minimally effective at best. Additionally, acetaminophen has been linked to liver damage, potentially resulting from glutathione depletion. Other side effects include:[13]

- bloody or black, tarry stools
- bloody or cloudy urine
- edema
- fever with or without chills (not present before treatment and not caused by the condition being treated)
- hypertension (high blood pressure)
- hypotension (low blood pressure)

- kidney failure
- liver toxicity
- nausea
- pain in the lower back and/or side (severe and/or sharp)
- pinpoint red spots on the skin
- skin rash, hives, or itching
- skin rashes
- sore throat (not present before treatment and not caused by the condition being treated)
- sores, ulcers, or white spots on the lips or in the mouth
- sudden decrease in the amount of urine
- unusual bleeding or bruising
- unusual tiredness or weakness
- vomiting
- yellow eyes or skin

In research milk thistle has been linked to elevated glutathione levels and, as a result, may help protect the liver. Supplementing with N-acetyle cysteine (NAC) may also be beneficial; hospitals use NAC to treat acetaminophen-induced liver damage.[14] Vitamin C may also be beneficial, as it appears to prolong the length of time acetaminophen stays in the body. Follow package directions for the specific nutritional and herbal products you choose.

The herb hibiscus should be avoided while taking acetaminophen because it may decrease levels of the drug in the body. Foods high in pectin such as cruciferous vegetables, apples, and preserves may interfere with acetaminophen absorption.[15] Due to potential liver side effects of acetaminophen and alcohol consumption, it is best to avoid alcohol while taking this drug.

TRAMADOL

Tramadol blocks the re-uptake of the neurotransmitter serotonin—an essential hormone needed to maintain healthy, balanced moods and health. Some of the side effects of tramadol include:[16]

- abdominal or stomach pain
- abnormal or decreased sensation of touch
- agitation
- anxiety
- blisters under the skin
- bloating
- blood in the urine
- blood pressure increased
- blurred vision
- change in walking and balance
- chest pain or discomfort
- chills
- constipation
- convulsions (seizures)
- cough
- darkened urine
- diarrhea
- difficult urination
- discouragement
- dizziness or lightheadedness when getting up from a lying or sitting position
- drowsiness
- dry mouth
- fainting
- fast heartbeat
- feeling of warmth
- feeling sad or empty
- feeling unusually cold
- fever
- frequent urge to urinate
- gaseous abdominal or stomach pain
- general feeling of discomfort or illness
- headache
- heart rate increase

- heartburn
- indigestion
- irregular heartbeat
- irritability
- itching of the skin
- joint pain
- loss of appetite
- loss of interest or pleasure
- loss of memory
- loss of strength or weakness
- muscle aches and pains
- nausea
- nervousness
- numbness and tingling of the face, fingers, or toes
- numbness, tingling, pain, or weakness in the hands or feet
- pain in the arms, legs, or lower back, especially pain in the calves or heels upon exertion
- pain or discomfort in the arms, jaw, back, or neck
- pain in the stomach, side, or abdomen, possibly radiating to the back
- pale bluish-colored or cold hands or feet
- recurrent fever
- redness of the face, neck, arms, and, occasionally, upper chest
- restlessness
- runny nose
- seeing, hearing, or feeling things that are not there
- severe cramping
- severe nausea
- severe redness, swelling, and itching of the skin
- shivering
- shortness of breath
- skin rash

- sleepiness or unusual drowsiness
- sore throat
- stuffy nose
- sweating
- sweats
- tiredness
- trembling and shaking of the hands or feet
- trouble concentrating
- trouble performing routine tasks
- unusual feeling of excitement
- weak or absent pulses in the legs
- weakness
- yellow eyes or skin

Alcohol may intensify the effects of the drug, so it is best to avoid drinking while taking tramadol.[17]

We might accept the serious side effects of many of these drugs if we knew they would cure us of what ails us, but the reality is that drugs don't cure disease; they mitigate symptoms. And in most cases they don't work much better—if at all better—than a placebo. According to Dr. Allen Roses, a scientist and the former global vice president of genetics at GlaxoSmithKline, "Most prescription medicines do not work on most people." He added, "The vast majority of drugs—more than 90 percent—only work on 30 to 50 percent of the people."[18]

Harvard University research found that approximately 50 percent of pharmaceutical drugs' effectiveness can actually be linked to the placebo effect, not the actual effectiveness of the medication. In the Harvard study, participants were given either a pain drug or a placebo. When either the drug or placebo was administered with the message that it is an "effective treatment," both had significantly better results. When the real drug was switched with the placebo, the results were nearly the same, provided that the message of the effective treatment accompanied the pills.[19]

It should be fairly clear by now that prescription drugs' effectiveness is much less than you may have believed. Much of their effectiveness can be attributed to the placebo effect or advertising or physician messaging that suggests that the drugs are effective. Additionally, when we refer to drugs as effective we simply mean they reduce symptoms. Sadly, no drug has ever cured arthritis. And considering the high cost, both financial and in terms of side effects, the minimal symptom improvement that pharmaceutical drugs sometimes offer is simply insufficient.

But if the story of arthritis were described in the classifications normally reserved for novels, it would not be a tragedy. No, it would be a romance. Like Barbara, many of my patients who learn about the benefits of a better diet complemented with natural supplements and remedies along with lifestyle changes not only experience symptom improvement but actually slow or halt disease progression and sometimes even reverse the effects of arthritis— no drug has ever done that. Many of these people, myself included, are so grateful for the quality of life that natural medicine helps restore that they become passionate about it. And there is plenty of reason to fall in love with natural medicine.

Consider that in a media release issued by the Orthomolecular Medicine News Service, entitled "Does Anybody Still Believe Slam Pieces on Dietary Supplements?" the organization reported, "the biological action of most prescription drugs can be duplicated with dietary supplements at far less cost and side effects . . ."[20] The nutrients, however, do not share the extensive list of side effects that accompany most prescription and OTC drugs, particularly in the category of pharmaceutically prepared analgesics. Twenty years ago medical professionals knew that nutrients could replace prescription drugs for treating disease.

As you'll soon discover, some groundbreaking advancements in the use of nutrition to treat arthritis were discovered nearly seventy years ago and then were largely forgotten or, worse, suppressed. And forget blaming bad genes for arthritis—pioneering research into a specific field known as nutrigenomics, the study of the effects of nutrition on the expression of DNA, found that certain nutrients formed compounds that could actually "turn off" the expression of so-called bad genes.[21] Whereas we once believed that our genes were comparable to ticking time bombs just waiting to go off, leading scientists and nutritionists now know that what we eat and how we live plays a much greater role in preventing or even reversing the effects of our genes than we ever imagined possible.

Over the next few chapters you'll learn more about the foods that harm, those that heal, the nutrient deficiencies that play causal roles in arthritis and how to address them, and the other nutrients and natural medicines that address the symptoms and speed healing of this serious condition. Although there is no such thing as a good time from which to suffer from serious conditions like arthritis, there has never been a more hopeful or empowering time to address this disease.

QUICK FACTS: AN ASPIRIN A DAY: FIVE THINGS YOU NEED TO KNOW

Many people take an aspirin a day to address pain and inflammation or simply because they believe it will prevent many health conditions. If you are among those taking aspirin daily, you should consider the drug's effects on your body and its essential nutrient stores. Here are five things you should consider:

1. Aspirin increases the loss of folic acid in urine while also reducing blood levels of folic acid. Because folic acid helps us deal with stress, keeps our immune system strong, and acts as a coenzyme to ensure the proper functioning of many biochemical reactions in our bodies, its depletion can cause a multitude of health problems. To counter

the lost folic acid, I usually recommend taking 400mcg of folic acid daily for arthritics taking aspirin.

2. Aspirin can cause gastrointestinal bleeding that causes loss of iron from the body. If continued over the long term, iron-deficiency anemia can result. Women, particularly during the menstrual years, may be vulnerable to anemia. Be sure to have your iron levels tested. Iron supplementation may be beneficial in cases where iron deficiency is confirmed with laboratory tests.

3. Aspirin may also deplete vitamin B12 in people with heart disease. The drug can also damage the stomach in some cases, an organ that plays a critical role in vitamin B12 absorption. Vitamin B12 is necessary for our energy levels, balanced moods, memory, and nervous system functions. Supplementary vitamin B12 may help address any deficiencies of this nutrient.

4. Aspirin may deplete vitamin C, which is required for bone and tooth formation, digestion, and blood cell formation. It helps accelerate wound healing, aids with the production of collagen that helps maintain skin's youthful elasticity, and is essential to helping us cope with stress. Supplementation of a few hundred milligrams of vitamin C daily may counter this depletion.

5. Aspirin has been shown to decrease blood levels of zinc. Zinc is required for properly digesting and utilizing carbohydrate foods like grains, vegetables, fruits, and sugars and protein foods like meat, eggs, and beans. The body needs carbohydrates to provide energy for all of its functions. Men typically have high zinc needs to support healthy prostate function. This essential mineral is necessary for the body to manufacture at least two hundred different enzymes needed for various aspects of metabolism and life. Our blood, bones, brain, heart, liver, and muscles also depend on adequate levels of this important mineral to function properly. Supplementing with 10mg of zinc daily may address these losses.

PAIN IS A FRIEND

Pain may feel like the worst enemy in your life, but it isn't; it's your body's way of trying to tell you something. Pain is the body's most effective warning signal that something is wrong. Pain is your friend—that is, if you listen to it instead of just trying to mask it or eliminate its sensations with pharmaceutical drugs. It may not be the friend you would like to show up on your doorstep, but it is a friend nonetheless. Learning to view pain in a different way will serve you well for the rest of your life. Pain is the means by which the intelligence of the body brings a problem situation to your attention. Does pain get your attention? Of course it does. Pain is also the body's attempt to heal itself. By masking the pain with OTC or prescription pain medications, you're simply avoiding the messages your body sends you.

It may seem impossible to accept that pain can be—and indeed is—your friend, particularly when it feels like it is ruining your life. But pain tells you when you're deficient in one or more nutrients, when you're overdoing some activity, when you aren't drinking enough water, when you're eating inflammatory foods, or when you may have an underlying infection that is causing the pain. Of course, you'll still need to play detective to get to the bottom of the specific reasons for your pain, but once you do, your body will thank you.

It's also important to realize that the current medical system typically involves prescribing the same drugs for arthritis, no matter who has the condition. But one person's arthritis may be quite different from another person's, particularly when you consider the source of the problems. One person may have a severe folate (vitamin B9) deficiency, whereas another person may be eating excessive inflammatory foods like French fries, diet soda, and sugary desserts. Another person, like Barbara, may have excessively high stress levels that cause a cascade of stress hormones to be released, which ultimately aggravate joint damage and cause pain. And there are many other potential causal factors for arthritis, which we will discuss throughout *Arthritis-Proof Your Life*. No one ever suffered from a pharmaceutical drug deficiency, but many have suffered from eating the wrong foods or eating insufficient nutrient-rich foods.

It's time to look at your body, diet, and lifestyle differently from how you may have in the past. Sure, it will take more work than popping a pill, but you'll actually be healing your body rather than just masking symptoms and creating a host of damaging drug side effects. In the next chapter we'll explore the dietary problems playing a significant role in the level of suffering you experience. And contrary to what you may have been told, arthritis is not just something that gets worse over time; there is a lot you can do to alleviate the pain and swelling of arthritis, not to mention the other symptoms, and get back to living life to its fullest.

2

Foods That Harm, Foods That Heal

FOODS ARE NOT SIMPLY for our enjoyment and nourishment; they're powerful healers in a vibrant multicolor disguise. Most people do not realize this fact because they're eating too many of the foods that harm and insufficient quantities of the foods that heal. Before you think that I'll have you on some starvation diet made up of only bland vegetables, keep reading—you're about to learn that the best healing remedies also taste fabulous. I certainly can't say that about any prescription medications.

THE INFLAMMATION CONNECTION

What's your favorite breakfast? Perhaps it is bacon, eggs, and coffee? Or maybe pancakes, sausage, and orange juice are more your style? Or maybe grabbing an Egg McMuffin, hash browns, and a coffee on your way to work is more your speed? Regard-less which of these breakfasts you might select, they all cause inflammation in the body—a serious problem for anyone suf-fering from arthritis.

Inflammation is the body's way of coping with an injury, infection, or an area of the body that needs healing attention. It signals that the body is sending white blood cells to the area to fight infection, oxygenated blood to repair damage, and other fluids to cushion any damaged cells. This process is perfectly normal and healthy. However, when inflammation lasts for long periods of time or when low-grade inflammation occurs in the body on an ongoing basis, it is essential you get it under control. That is one of the reasons why injured joints tend to be more vulnerable to disorders like arthritis: the damaged area can be vulnerable to further damage and inflammation over time.

Yet most of our everyday foods, not just those we select for breakfast, actually cause inflammation and aggravate arthritis. The Standard American Diet, aptly shortened to SAD, is high in sugars and refined carbs, trans fats or hydrogenated fats, and chemical food additives, to name a few of the inflammatory food ingredients.

THE HEALING POWER OF FOOD

You've heard the old adage "you are what you eat." Nothing could be more true when it comes to dealing with illness. If you are suffering from pain and inflammation it's time for a close examination of your diet, along with some tweaks to help you restore great health.

The Sugar Correlation

If I told you there is a white powdery substance that is extremely damaging to your joints and tissues you probably wouldn't think

I was talking about sugar. But increasingly research shows that sugar causes inflammation in the body.

When I tell most people about sugar's correlation to arthritis, they tell me it doesn't apply to them because they don't eat sweets or a high-sugar diet. If you think the research doesn't apply to you, consider that the Standard American Diet is a high-sugar diet. Sugar is hidden in virtually all processed, packaged, and prepared foods. Industrial sugar processing has increased individual consumption of this lethal sweetener by twenty-five *times* over the last century. According to the US Department of Agriculture (USDA), per capita consumption of caloric sweeteners such as sucrose (table sugar) and high-fructose corn syrup increased 43 pounds, or 39 percent, between 1959 and 2000.[1] The average American consumes about 152 pounds of sugar annually, the equivalent of fifty-two teaspoons of added sugars every day. This is over and above the naturally occurring sugars present in fruit, vegetables, grains, and legumes, which provide more than enough sugar in our daily diets. Compare that with our ancestors' diet a century ago: they ate only about five pounds of sugar each year. This excessive amount sugar not only aggravates existing inflammation but also causes inflammation in the joints and throughout the body.

Soda is one of the worst sources of sugar, containing seven to eleven teaspoons per can and much more than that for the supersized beverages now sold at many fast food restaurants. Sugar is insidious in our diet, hiding in many unsuspected places, including condiments, meat, French fries, and even in some salt. It's shocking but true.

You don't have to give up all of your favorite foods to significantly reduce your sugar consumption. By taking charge of your food choices, reading labels on packages, avoiding fast foods and most restaurant menu items, and reducing your consumption of alcohol and canned or bottled beverages, you will cut out many pounds of sugar annually. Be aware that sugar hides in many packaged and prepared foods. Look for any ingredient that contains "-ose," such as glucose, high-fructose corn syrup, fructose, dextrose, maltose, and so forth. Even natural sweeteners like honey, pure maple syrup, agave nectar, and barley malt are high in sugars and should be used sparingly. Treat your sweet tooth occasionally with delicious fresh fruit, and see how much better you feel once the sugar monkey is off your back.

Additionally, sweeten your coffee or tea with stevia, or *Stevia rebaudiana*, which is a natural herb that tastes sweet but doesn't actually contain sugar molecules. As a result it doesn't affect blood sugar levels or cause inflammation in the body and is therefore a good option for healthy joints and a healthy body. It is naturally between three hundred and one thousand times sweeter than sugar, depending on whether you're using the whole herb or the liquid extract. I personally find liquid stevia has the best taste and least aftertaste, but I have found powdered ones that are excellent as well.

You can also switch other sugars in your diet to the naturally sweet herb stevia. Replace sugar on your oatmeal or in your cereal with stevia, which is available in many forms, including liquid extract, powdered extract, or powdered herb. Be aware that some manufacturers of the powdered extract of stevia include other sweeteners alongside the herb, so these products are best avoided.

Because stevia is naturally sweet, you won't need much to sweeten your tea, coffee, or other foods and beverages; just a few drops is sufficient. The powder usually comes with what looks like a doll-sized spoon because that's all you'll need for most beverages.

Baking with stevia poses some challenges because, other than sweetening, it doesn't have the same chemical properties of sugar, such as caramelizing when heated or becoming chewy in cookies. Also, because you need to use so little stevia it may throw off the traditional dry-to-wet ingredient ratio if you try to substitute stevia. So you may need to experiment a bit with your recipes or try some recipes that were specifically designed with stevia as the sweetener.

SIX REASONS TO AVOID LIKE THE PLAGUE
HIGH-FRUCTOSE CORN SYRUP

If you take a look at most candy, cereal, bread, frozen food, yogurt, baby food, granola bars, salad dressings, crackers, condiments, or other processed food packages, you're sure to see high-fructose corn syrup (HFCS) on the ingredients list. It might even be easy to equate commonality with safety, assuming that that if HFCS really was damaging to your health, surely the Food and Drug Administration (FDA) would ban it, right? Wrong. Just because it has the name "corn" in it (which most people equate with a healthy vegetable) combined with the fact that it is found almost everywhere doesn't make it safe to eat.

The average American currently consumes fifty-five pounds of HFCS every year, which is a higher per capita consumption than in any other country.[2] If you're currently consuming HFCS (and most people are eating plentiful amounts without even realizing it), you'll probably want to reconsider after reading the six reasons to avoid it like the plague:

Chronic inflammation: HFCS irritates the gut lining until it causes small perforations, allowing partially digested food, fecal matter, and harmful bacteria to cross the intestinal wall directly into the bloodstream. The result: inflammation and an overactive immune system caused by the body's own immune system attacking these substances it perceives as foreign invaders. And what feeds the joints and soft tissue in the body? Blood. So the same immune system attacks can occur in the joints and soft tissues of the body, resulting in conditions like rheumatoid arthritis or fibromyalgia.[3]

Energy depletion: Sugar found in HFCS requires higher amounts of energy to be absorbed by the gut than do other types of sugar. Each molecule requires two molecules of phosphorus from our body's ATP, which is our body's energy currency. The result is energy depletion. The cells in your joints and tissues lack the energy they need to maintain healthy joints or heal damaged ones.[4]

Obesity: Because HFCS requires little to no digestion, it is quickly absorbed into the bloodstream. As a result, the sugar causes rapid spikes in insulin production, which is the body's fat storage hormone. Not only does your appetite increase, so does your weight. It's no surprise that the high consumption of high fructose corn syrup is linked to obesity.[5] Further, obesity results in a much higher impact on the joints, which can aggravate arthritis.

Diabetes: Research at the University of Southern California and Oxford University found that HFCS is linked with diabetes, which may explain the rapidly growing rates of diabetes. Their research showed that HFCS consumption is linked to a 20 percent higher prevalence of diabetes in those who consume HFCS than those who don't.[6]

Fatty liver disease: Consumption of HFCS has also been linked to fatty liver disease.[7] The liver must metabolize HFCS, and this puts a tremendous strain on this already hard-working organ and makes you vulnerable to weight gain and obesity, among other conditions.

Increased blood pressure and heart disease risk: A study published in the *Journal of the American Society of Nephrology* found that even people who eat an otherwise healthy diet but consume HFCS are at risk of an increase in blood pressure by up to 32 percent. The study, conducted at the University of Colorado, found that the inflammation caused by HFCS leads to inflammation in the bloodstream, which causes the blood vessel walls to tighten, resulting in blood pressure increases.[8]

Artificial Sweeteners

Because sugar is so damaging to health, you may be tempted to switch to artificial sweeteners, or you may have already bought into the marketing claims. There are a few different types of artificial sweeteners, including NutraSweet, Splenda (saccharin), and AminoSweet (aspartame), but due to their many negative health effects, they are all best avoided. Research links these nasty substances to many serious health conditions, including pain and inflammation—both unwanted symptoms for arthritics.

In a study released in *Nature: the International Weekly Journal of Science*, researchers linked the ingestion of artificial sweeteners to increased blood sugar levels (an early indicator of type 2 diabetes). Additionally, the study found that consumption of commonly used non-caloric artificial sweeteners disrupt the microbial balance in the gut, which, as you'll learn, is a factor in the development of arthritis.[9]

Bad Carb, Good Carb

Sugar isn't the only problem. Most people choose the wrong types of carbohydrates, or carbs, like white potatoes, white rice, and white flour and foods made with it. Some of the bad carb foods include pastries, doughnuts, candies, cakes, white bread, "multigrain" bread (which is actually mostly white flour with a handful of grains added to it), and whole-wheat bread (which also tends to be largely white flour with a small amount of whole wheat added to it).

These foods have a similar effect to sugar on the body. They cause wild blood sugar fluctuations that result in low-grade inflammation anywhere in the body. Does that mean you need to give up all of your favorite carbs? No, of course not. Many breads, pastries, cakes and other foods can be made with whole-grain flour that does not have the same inflammatory effect on your body.

And instead of white rice or white potatoes, choose whole grains like brown rice, buckwheat, millet, oats, quinoa, or wild rice. They can be made into delicious whole-grain dishes with chopped vegetables and spices or cooked and made into hearty salads with the addition of chopped fruits, vegetables, and seasonings.

Great Grains for an Anti-Inflammatory Diet

There are many grains that are, not only nutritionally superior to white rice but also make delicious additions to your diet. All of the following grains are free of gluten, a type of protein found in many grains and foods made with them, particularly wheat, rye, and barley. Many arthritics are sensitive to gluten (I'll explain more later), so it's a good idea to choose gluten-free grains like the following to add to your diet.

BROWN RICE

Unlike white rice, brown rice is high in fiber and vitamin E. Vitamin E is essential for healthy lubrication of joints and a balanced immune system as well as many other critical functions in your body. During the processing of brown rice into white, these nutrients are largely lost. Brown rice also contains high amounts of the minerals manganese, magnesium, and selenium as well as tryptophan, which helps with sleep. Selenium helps ward off cancer. Brown rice can easily replace white rice in almost any recipe—soups, stews, stir-fries, and even to make a dairy-free milk substitute.

BUCKWHEAT

The name is a bit misleading. Buckwheat is not related to wheat and is both wheat- and gluten-free. It's not even technically a grain but rather a seed that's a relative of rhubarb. It is high in fiber, manganese, magnesium, tryptophan, and copper. Research shows that the regular consumption of buckwheat reduces the incidence of high blood pressure or high cholesterol. The combination of vitamin C and the flavonoid rutin give buckwheat its ability to prevent blood clumping and to keep blood moving smoothly through blood vessels, which helps to ensure adequate oxygenation of tissues and joints.

MILLET

Similar in texture to couscous, millet is high in manganese, phosphorus, tryptophan, and magnesium. Phosphorus is a key component of ATP, your body's energy currency. ATP helps ensure that your body has the energy it needs for every function. Tryptophan is the amino acid that helps your body make melatonin, which in turn helps you sleep like a baby at night. Magnesium helps to regulate the nervous system and pain signals, making adequate amounts essential for arthritics and those suffering from fibromyalgia.

OATS

Oats help stabilize blood sugar and lower cholesterol and are high in protein and fiber. Oats are available in many forms, including instant, steel cut, rolled, bran, groats, flakes, and flour. The best options are the less refined ones like steel cut, rolled, flakes, and bran. Oat flour is an excellent substitute for wheat flour in baking recipes. It is also a good source of minerals like manganese, selenium, magnesium, and the sleep aid tryptophan, which can help improve sleep quality, an issue for many people suffering from pain.

QUINOA

Quinoa, a staple of the ancient Incas who revered it as sacred, is not a true grain; rather, it is the seed of an herb. Unlike most grains, quinoa is a complete protein and is high in iron, magnesium, B-vitamins, and fiber. In studies quinoa is a proven aid for migraine sufferers and, like most whole grains, lessens the risk for heart disease. It also contains the building blocks for superoxide dismutase, an important antioxidant that helps protect the energy centers of your cells from free radical damage, thereby ensuring that your body's healing functions have adequate energy supplies to maintain healthy joints and tissues.

WILD RICE

Like millet and quinoa, wild rice is not truly a grain; it's actually a type of aquatic grass seed native to the United States and Canada. It tends to be a bit pricier than other grains, but its high content of protein and nutty flavor make wild rice worth every penny. It's an excellent choice for people who have gluten or wheat sensitivities, as many arthritics do (we'll discuss food sensitivities in arthritis momentarily). At eighty-three calories per half cup of cooked rice, wild rice also has a lower caloric content than many grains, and it is high in fiber. Add wild rice to soups, stews, salads, and pilaf. It's important to note that wild rice is black. There are many blends of white and wild rice, which primarily consist of refined white rice; be sure to use only real wild rice, not the blends.

What Exactly Is Gluten?

Gluten is a set of specific proteins found in some grains like wheat, barley, spelt, kamut, rye, and others as well as baked goods, cereals, seasonings, and other foods made from these grains.

Some but not all arthritics have a sensitivity or full-blown inflammatory reaction when they eat foods that contain gluten, which may be perfectly healthy for other people. Ask your doctor or nutritionist to test you for gluten intolerance to determine whether you should avoid gluten-containing grains. Many physicians do not recognize gluten intolerance as a disease condition although there is a great deal of research to support it; as a result, many doctors will not conduct the tests for it. Try to choose a holistically minded physician or nutritionist. All of the grains I discussed above in the Great Grains for an Anti-Inflammatory Diet section are gluten-free; however, be aware that oats can sometimes be contaminated with wheat and are not gluten-free unless the package indicates that they are certified gluten-free oats.

In addition to the above whole grains, here are some of the best gluten-free flour options you can choose instead of white or wheat flour in your baking.

Amaranth flour has a unique and earthy flavor and is high in fiber and protein. It is neither a grain nor a grass but is actually a plant that is related to spinach and Swiss chard. The plant produces flowers that have a large number of seeds, which are ground into amaranth flour. It is rich in the amino acid lysine, which is often used to treat viruses and infections, and these may be a factor in arthritis. Additionally, it is an excellent source of iron, calcium, and vitamin E.

Arrowroot is a starch or flour made from the ground roots of the plant *Maranta arundinacea*. It is easily digested, light and delicate, and highly nutritious. Arrowroot starch or flour contains calcium and trace minerals. According to Bob's Red Mills website, when Europeans first encountered the Arawak natives, the indigenous people informed them that the food was called *aru aru*, which means "meal of meals," representing the value the natives placed on the ground root. Because the flour is so light, it adds a lightness to gluten-free baked goods and pastries.

Brown rice is frequently eaten as part of a gluten-free diet, but it is also available ground to use in gluten-free baking. Brown rice and brown rice flour are high in minerals such as magnesium, manganese, and selenium, and it is higher in fiber and vitamin E than white rice. The flour has the denser quality of whole-grain flour, making it good used for whole-grain bread baking. It is usually paired with lighter gluten-free flours such as arrowroot or tapioca for lighter baked goods.

Buckwheat's name is a bit misleading. As I mentioned above, it is not related to wheat at all and is gluten-free. Instead, it is a relative of rhubarb and is high in tryptophan, which converts into the sound-sleep hormone melatonin in the body to help ensure a deeper, restorative sleep, which can help boost healing in arthritics. It is also high in copper, magnesium, manganese, and, of course, fiber.

Chickpea flour adds a sweet, slightly bean-y taste along with plentiful amounts of fiber to baked goods. High in protein, iron, and molybdenum, this flour is usually combined with other flours to avoid excessively bean-y tasting breads or pastries.

Coconut flour is a great high-fiber and high-protein option that is great for gluten-free baking; however, it does not perform similarly to other types of flour when used in most recipes. It usually requires some practice and finessing to make it work for many baked goods. Ideally, simply choose a good coconut flour cookbook or recipe that has been designed with coconut in mind.

Millet flour is a lesser-used gluten-free flour, but I think it should be used more frequently because it is high in fiber, delicious, and packed with nutrients like magnesium, tryptophan, manganese, and phosphorus. The latter mineral aids the body in energy production. Millet flour is derived from the seeds of a grass that is closely related to sorghum. When used in baking it tends to impart a light quality.

Oats are gluten-free but because they are frequently contaminated with wheat while growing or being processed, it is important to select certified gluten-free varieties, particularly if you have a severe intolerance or allergy to gluten. Oat flour has a naturally sweet taste and imparts a delicious flavor and a light texture to breads and other baked goods. Oats are high in B vitamins, iron, calcium, fiber, and vitamin E.

Quinoa (pronounced keen-WAH) is an ancient grain (technically a seed) that was originally used by the Incas who revered it as sacred. Considering that the seed is a complete protein—something few grains can claim—it is easy to see why the Incas valued it so highly, as they likely depended on it to avoid serious nutritional deficiencies. Quinoa flour is one of the most nutritious due to the high protein content as well as zinc, iron, B vitamins, calcium, phosphorus, potassium, magnesium, and manganese content.

Sorghum flour (also known as milo flour) comes from whole kernels from the sorghum plant. It is high in protein and has a mellow taste and light texture, making baked goods made with it less dense. It contains niacin, calcium, potassium, and phosphorus.

Tapioca flour is made from cassava root that has been boiled, dried, and ground into a flour. Although it does not contain any protein it has a small amount of folate and some iron, calcium, magnesium, manganese, selenium, zinc, and copper. It has a light texture and is frequently used to make baked goods lighter or less dense and to tone down stronger-flavored flours.

Teff flour is milled from the North African grain known as teff. It is the smallest grain in the world. It has a unique and slightly nutty taste that imparts a delicious flavor and lots of nutrition to baked goods. Like quinoa, it is a complete protein and is also high in lysine, calcium, copper, and iron.

TWELVE TIPS FOR FOOL-PROOF GLUTEN-FREE BAKING

Anyone who has ever tried to apply the principles of traditional wheat baking to gluten-free baking quickly learns the hard way that there are few similarities. I've been baking gluten-free for several years and here are some of the things I learned that I wish I had known when I started:

1. Gluten-free baked goods do not require kneading. Kneading is the means by which gluten in wheat-based baking is activated. Because there is no gluten in grains used in gluten-free baking, you can skip

this step altogether, making gluten-free baking much easier than wheat-based baking.

2. Gluten acts as glue and imparts elasticity to hold traditional baked goods together and allow bakers to work with the dough, cutting or molding it into different shapes. In the absence of this gluey substance, baked goods tend to crumble unless some other form of binder is added.

3. Not all gluten-free binding agents were created equally. Some of the typical binding agents used in gluten-free baking include eggs (which you'll obviously want to avoid if you're vegan or suspect a food sensitivity), xanthan gum, guar gum, and flax or chia seeds (when mixed with water or other liquid ingredients). Even flours like arrowroot and tapioca offer some binding properties, albeit less than the other binding agents, when they are baked.

4. Although xanthan is frequently touted as a healthy and safe option, I can hardly support that claim. Xanthan, or xanthan gum as it is also known, is a carbohydrate secreted by the bacteria known as *Xanthomonas campestris*. These bacteria, which cause disease in plants, are mixed with fermented sugars, which are usually sourced from corn or sugar beets, lactose (the sugar present in milk), wheat, or soy to form a gummy substance. Not only is this source likely to be manufactured from genetically modified ingredients; there is also the possibility of contamination if wheat is used in the process. Most of my clients who have used xanthan in their baking or eaten prepared foods containing it find that they are bloated, gaseous, and experience abdominal cramping within hours of eating foods containing this laboratory-concocted ingredient.

5. Whereas wheat, rye, and barley contain gluten, as you learned earlier, there are many other excellent flour options available for your gluten-free baking.

6. Although gluten-free flours can largely be used interchangeably, they do change the flavor, texture, moisture, and density of the finished baked good. Coconut flour is an excellent example: it is highly

absorbent of moisture and can throw off the dry-to-wet ratios in most recipes. So unless you're working with a recipe created for use with coconut flour, you might want to wait until you're experienced with gluten-free baking to start using this flour.

7. You'll probably want to use a blend of flours to obtain the consistency of baked goods you'd like. Flours like brown rice, buckwheat, sorghum, millet, oat, quinoa, teff, almond, hazelnut, chestnut, chickpea, soy, and coconut tend to increase the density of a finished baked good (similar to whole wheat). Flours like arrowroot, corn, potato, white rice, sweet rice, sorghum, or tapioca tend to offer softness to the texture of baked goods (similar to white flour). You'll notice that sorghum appears twice. That's intentional, as it can add lightness or density, depending on how it is milled. The package usually indicates "whole sorghum flour" or "refined sorghum flour" or something else to indicate how refined it is. Keep in mind that foods made with some of these flours, such as corn, potato, white rice, and sweet rice, are quite similar to white flour in that they can cause blood sugar levels to spike, so beware of overusing these options, as they can aggravate joint pain and inflammation.

8. You can increase the amount of protein in your gluten-free baking by choosing options like almond, hazelnut, buckwheat, and quinoa flour. Ground almonds or hazelnuts are the same as almond or hazelnut flour, respectively. Quinoa flour has a bold flavor, and you might want to use it in moderation, as it imparts a strong flavor to any baked goods made with it.

9. Although it is fine to use some flours like arrowroot, tapioca, and sweet rice to add softness to your baking, cut these flours with other types to prevent the final product from being gummy.

10. Choose a gluten-free baking powder, as most commercial baking powders tend to be a source of gluten and can be a problem for those individuals who are highly sensitive to gluten.

11. Puréed fruit, such as applesauce, can add moisture to gluten-free baking, preventing it from drying out.

12. For ideal bread baking you'll want a thinner texture of batter than you normally would use with wheat breads. Cookie batter can spread quickly once it is heated, so you may want to chill it first.

Why the Wrong Fats Are a Serious Threat

Most packaged, processed, or prepared foods contain these incredibly harmful fats in the form of fried foods, shortening, lard, and even margarine, which many people believe is healthy. Margarine is actually a toxic chemical that the body does not recognize as food; in addition to clogging arteries, it contributes to arthritic symptoms and worsens inflammation.

The typical diet, if it contains any healthy essential fatty acids, usually includes fats from meat and poultry or from nuts and seeds. Most diets are high in essential fatty acids known as omega 6s. Although these fats are healthy in a ratio of one-to-one or even two-to-one of omega 6s to omega 3s, another essential fatty acid that the body must get from food, most people eat a twenty-to-one ratio. This excess worsens and even causes inflammation in the body. Omega 6 fatty acids are found in the highest concentrations in corn, sunflower, and safflower oils as well as from the meat of animals that eat a diet high in these fats. Eating too many omega 6 fatty acids in contrast to omega 3 fatty acids will produce substances in the body that will trigger or worsen existing inflammation. Yet that is exactly what the Standard American Diet contains: too many omega 6s and not enough omega 3 fatty acids.

Consuming oils like corn oil, safflower oil, sunflower oil, or vegetable oil, which is usually a combination of corn, canola, and/or safflower oil, along with eating the meat of animals fed these fats in their diets, can worsen inflammation in the body, aggravate arthritic pain, and negate the beneficial effects of healthy oils. Although many people know that fish—not the battered and fried variety—can be a healthier food choice thanks to its omega 3 fatty acid content, few people realize that if you eat a salad in which the dressing is made of one of the above-mentioned oils along with a piece of fatty fish, the oil in the salad will undo the benefits of eating the fish. Another example is tuna fish or sardines made into tuna salad or served on a sandwich alongside mayonnaise: the mayonnaise and the oils in the bread will counter any positive effects of eating the fish and lengthen or, worse, prevent the full healing of joint injuries or aggravate existing joint inflammation in the body.

Also, be sure to avoid peanuts, peanut oil, and foods cooked in peanut oil because they tend to contain many aflatoxins (mold-like substances) that aggravate joints and tissues, causing pain and inflammation.

THE JOY OF FISH OILS

There are many foods that are scientifically proven, all-natural anti-inflammatories. The most popular are foods that contain omega 3 fatty acids. Omega 3s are found in fatty cold water fish like salmon, mackerel, sardines, anchovies, and tuna. In the body omega 3s convert into hormone-like substances that decrease inflammation.

According to Dr. Alfred D. Steinberg, an arthritis expert at the National Institute of Health, fish oil is an anti-inflammatory agent. Fish oil acts directly on the immune system by suppressing 40 to 55 percent of the release of cytokines, compounds known to destroy joints.

There are many studies demonstrating that eating moderate amounts of fish or taking fish oil reduces inflammation, particularly for arthritis. Dr. Joel M. Kremer, MD, conducted a double-blind study of thirty-three patients with multiple swollen and tender joints, fatigue, and morning stiffness lasting for more than a half hour. When they took fish oil capsules for fourteen weeks their symptoms improved. Joint tenderness improved by more than one-third, and the participants were free of fatigue for over two and a half hours longer each day.

Dr. Kremer found that fish oils suppressed the body's production of leukotriene B4, the main inflammatory substance in the body and the one considered largely responsible for arthritic symptoms. He observed that the lower the production of leukotriene B4, the fewer the number of tender joints.

Another study had similar results with fish oil and found that leukotrienes lessened within one month of supplementation with fish oil. When a person discontinues taking fish oil, leukotriene production increases again within one month, so it is important to continue eating fatty fish or supplementing with fish oil over the long-term to continue reaping the health benefits.

Dr. Kremer suggests that the longer a person continues taking fish oil, the more rapid and intense the improvements. The daily amount used in the study was the equivalent of eating a seven-ounce serving of salmon or two cans of sardines per day.

Eating fish oil or supplementing with fish oil capsules daily can go a long way toward restoring your joint health and alleviating joint or body-wide inflammation. Keep in mind that it takes more fish oil to reduce arthritis than to prevent arthritis or maintain joint health.

OTHER SOURCES OF BENEFICIAL OMEGA 3S

Other foods with high amounts of omega 3 fatty acids include flaxseeds and flaxseed oil, walnut oil and raw walnuts, and dark leafy greens like spinach and kale. But do not heat or cook with flaxseed oil; it is best reserved for salad dressings or as a topping for steamed vegetables or baked potatoes. Walnut oil, although a bit pricy, is an excellent cooking oil or base for salad dressings as well as an excellent way to add more omega 3 fatty oils to your diet.

WHEN SMOKE GETS IN YOUR EYES

It's not just the misplaced ratio of essential fatty acids that pre-disposes us to inflammation; it is also the quality of the oils we eat. All oils have different smoke points—the temperature above which the oil begins to smoke and is no longer healthy to eat. When oils smoke, their delicate essential oils become damaged, causing inflammation and, in some cases, also becoming car-cinogenic. Because of this, oils that have extremely low smoke points, such as flaxseed oil, should never be heated. Olive oil smokes at about 320 degrees Fahrenheit, whereas macadamia nut oil reaches its smoke point around 413 degrees Fahrenheit. Like olive oil, walnut oil has a smoke point of about 320 degrees Fahrenheit and should therefore be used on low to medium heat. Most oils sold in grocery stores, however, have been heated to extremely high temperatures during their processing and packaging, even before you get them home and begin to cook with them. These overheated or rancid oils no longer sup-port joint health and actually create inflammation in the body; extra-virgin olive oil is the exception. Some grocery stores are moving to refrigerated, cold-pressed virgin oils, but this is still fairly rare. Most health food stores offer healthier, refrigerated, cold-pressed oils.

Fried Foods

I probably don't need to explain that fried foods such as French fries, onion rings, potato chips, and nachos cause inflamma-tion. Most people know these items are not healthy choices and have no redeeming health quality because the oils used in frying are frequently heated to excessive temperatures, often before they are even bottled for cooking and then again during the frying process. The oils are then used over and over again. When these oils are heated past their smoke point or are reused on a regular basis, they become inflammation-causing oils. What you might not realize, however, is that these foods contribute to arthritis and fibromyalgia and need to be eliminated from your diet.

Milk Does the Body Harm

Forget the slogan promoted by dairy marketing bureaus that "milk does the body good." Milk is highly inflammatory, and people with arthritis should avoid it. Research even links dairy products with the formation of arthritis. In one study on rabbits, scientist Richard Panush was able to produce inflamed joints in the study animals by switching their water to milk. In another study scientists observed more than a 50 percent reduction in the pain and swelling of arthritis when participants eliminated milk and dairy products from their diet.

Not only are the naturally present hormones in cow's milk stronger than human hormones, but the animals are also routinely given steroids and other hormones to plump them up and increase milk production. These hormones can negatively impact humans' delicate hormonal balance, resulting in a condition known as estrogen dominance, in which estrogen levels are excessive in relation to progesterone—two naturally present hormones in the body. When estrogen levels remain high, inflammation typically results. Additionally, because most commercial feed for cows contains all sorts of ingredients that include genetically modified (GM) corn, GM soy, animal products, chicken manure, cottonseed, pesticides, and antibiotics, the milk produced by these animals is anything but a health food. Most milk and dairy products now contain something known as rBST. BST is a hormone known as bovine somatotropin that is normally present in dairy products, but rBST is a genetically modified version (the "r" stands for recombinant) of the hormone and was developed in a laboratory using genetically engineered *E. coli* bacteria.

Forget what you've heard about dairy products being the best source of calcium. Research shows that the countries whose citizens consume the most dairy products have the highest incidence of osteoporosis, contrary to what dairy marketing boards will have you believe. Plant-based sources of calcium are far more digestible and absorbable than calcium found in dairy products. Most milk is homogenized, which denatures the milk's proteins, making it harder to digest. As a result, many peoples' bodies react to these proteins as though they are "foreign invaders," causing their immune systems to overreact. And as you'll learn later in this book, foods that cause the immune system to overreact are a serious problem in arthritis, particularly rheumatoid arthritis.

There are many delicious alternatives to milk; however, don't expect them to taste like milk—they don't. Each milk alternative has its own unique and delicious flavor. Experiment with them to find which ones you enjoy most. You can add them to your coffee or tea, replace milk in baking, or drink them on their own. Most health food stores carry almond milk, rice milk, coconut milk, hemp milk, soy milk, or combinations of plant-based milks. I don't recommend soy milk for people with arthritis, as many arthritics have an undiagnosed soy sensitivity that they might not even be aware of. I'll share more information about food sensitivities later in this chapter.

Undoubtedly, when I tell people about the perils of dairy products they ask, "Where will I get my calcium?" We've been duped into believing that dairy products equate with calcium. As stated above, although dairy products tend to be high in calcium, the body does not absorb it effectively, and worse than that, it creates excessive inflammation and disease. Fortunately there are many excellent sources of calcium that are easy to digest and the body can absorb them easily. Here are some of the best sources.

Top Calcium-Rich Foods (per 100 grams/4 ounces):[10]

beet greens	119mg
broccoli	103mg
collard (leaves)	250mg
collard (stems)	203mg
dandelion greens	187mg
fennel	100mg
kale (leaves)	249mg
kale (stems)	179mg
mustard greens	183mg
parsley	203mg
pepper, red hot	130mg
seaweed, agar	567mg
seaweed, dulse	296mg
turnip greens	246mg
watercress	151mg
chickpeas	150mg
mung bean sprouts	118mg
almonds	234mg
brazil nuts*	186mg
hazelnuts (filberts)*	209mg
sesame seeds	1,160mg
sunflower seeds	120mg

SUMMARY OF THE MAIN FOODS
THAT CAUSE INFLAMMATION

Everyday foods like bacon, eggs, coffee, and dairy products cause inflammation. That might not sound like a big deal, but it's important to realize that arthritis as well as most other chronic conditions such as cancer, diabetes, and obesity have been linked to inflammation. Actually, low-grade inflammation is a factor in most health issues. And when you suffer from a pain disorder like arthritis, you better believe that inflammatory foods will aggravate the condition.

Many common foods in the Standard American Diet can cause or exacerbate inflammation in the body, but the following twelve top my list of most inflammatory foods.

The "3 Ps"–processed, packaged, or prepared foods. And yes, fast food is atop the list of inflammatory foods thanks to its harmful oils, sugar and artificial sweeteners, food additives, and a whole host of nasty ingredients.

Hydrogenated and trans fats found in margarine, shortening, lard, or products made with them. That includes many baked goods, cookies, pies, buns. Of course, there are healthier alternatives to these baked goods, but most grocery stores and bakeries are using these harmful ingredients.

Red meat (this does not include red-fleshed, wild-caught fish). I'm not suggesting you have to go vegan or vegetarian here, although a plant-based diet tends to be much lower in inflammatory substances, but meat and poultry cause inflammation, so make them the background of your meals, not the main dish.

Fried foods (French fries, onion rings, potato chips, nachos, hamburgers, etc.). I think these items speak for themselves. I doubt anyone thinks they are healthy.

White sugar and sweets, including soft drinks and sweetened juices. Newer research is showing that sugar is one of the most addictive substances you can use. It's also highly inflammatory. No, you don't need to eliminate sugar and sweets altogether–simply reduce your consumption and choose fruit as your "go to" food when you're craving something sweet.

High-fructose corn syrup-containing foods. High-fructose corn syrup is hidden in most foods. Because it has such a significant link to inflammation, I've included a whole text box on the topic. See Six Reasons to Avoid Like the Plague High-Fructose Corn Syrup, which I discussed earlier.

Synthetic sweeteners (Nutrasweet, Splenda, saccharin, aspartame, AminoSweet, etc.). Research links these nasty substances to many serious health conditions. I avoid them like the plague as well.

Food additives (colors, flavor enhancers, stabilizers, preservatives, etc.). Some of the more popular additives include sulfites, benzoates, and colors named FD&C #. . . . Unfortunately many foods that children consume are loaded with these harmful, toxic ingredients.

Dairy products (yogurt, ice cream, cottage cheese, butter, cheese, etc.). The reasons dairy products are inflammatory are too lengthy to list here, but today's dairy products are packed with hormones, antibiotics, and other harmful ingredients, so avoid them as much as possible.

Wheat products. Wheat is highly acid forming and inflammatory in the body. Most wheat is heavily sprayed with toxic pesticides that stay in the grain after it has been milled. These pesticides can cause or aggravate inflammation.

Other gluten-containing grains. Gluten is found in most grains and is highly inflammatory in susceptible individuals. Although not everyone with arthritis or fibromyalgia is sensitive to gluten, most are. Choose grains or seeds like amaranth, buckwheat, quinoa, or millet for your baking.

Alcohol. High in sugar and a burden to the liver, which works to eliminate inflammation by-products from the blood, alcohol makes the top twelve inflammatory foods list. It is best eliminated or minimally used.

By now it may be obvious that the Standard American Diet (SAD) does not support health, and it certainly doesn't support joint health. Try reducing your consumption of these foods with the goal of eliminating them completely. Don't worry: there are many other delicious foods you can eat. And with a few simple ingredient substitutions, you'll find you can enjoy many of your favorite foods.

The Meat of the Problem

Red meat and hormone- and antibiotic-laced poultry are well-established causes of inflammation in the body. I'm not suggesting you become vegan or vegetarian to address arthritis, although a plant-based diet tends to be much less inflammatory; rather, it is wise to reduce the amount of processed meat like deli meats, bacon, sausages, and other meat products, particularly those that contain artificial ingredients and preservatives, as they are inflammatory additions. The World Health Organization (WHO) has even declared these foods to be carcinogens. If you eat meat, it is best to choose organic or hormone- and antibiotic-free options.

Here are a few reasons to significantly reduce the amount of meat you eat if you are suffering from arthritis or fibromyalgia.

- Meat contains the type of fat that stimulates the production of inflammatory agents in the body.
- Bacon, pork, and beef especially stimulate the inflammatory process.
- In many people it produces arthritis flare-ups and allergic reactions.
- Processed meats, particularly cured meats such as bacon, ham, hot dogs, and cold cuts, contain preservatives and other chemicals that trigger inflammation in some individuals.

There are many benefits of eating a plant-based diet. In my twenty-five years of experience as a nutritionist I've found that a plant-based diet is highly effective for treating arthritis and fibromyalgia. That doesn't mean you have to swear off meat or chicken completely; it simply means you should reduce the amount of these foods in your diet while adding more vegetables, fruits, legumes, and gluten-free grains. Research supports the effectiveness of a plant-based diet for arthritis. Studies have demonstrated that feeding a high-fat diet like the Standard American Diet to animals susceptible to autoimmune diseases increases the severity of rheumatoid arthritis.[11] Conversely, studies also show that a vegetarian, gluten-free diet significantly improved symptoms of rheumatoid arthritis.[12] As you learned earlier, the Standard American Diet, with its heavy reliance on fatty foods like meat, cheeses, and fried foods, tends to be highly inflammatory, whereas vegetarian diets tend to have a higher portion of anti-inflammatory effects.

Jean Carper recounts a study in her book *Food: Your Miracle Medicine* that demonstrates the benefits of a vegetarian diet for people suffering from joint damage: "Jens Kjeldsen-Kragh, M.D., of the Institute of Immunology and Rheumatology at the National Rheumatism Hospital of Oslo, found that switching to a vegetarian diet resulted in better grip strength and much less pain, joint swelling and tenderness and morning stiffness in about 90 percent of a group of arthritic subjects, compared with the control group eating an ordinary diet. The subjects noticed improvement within a month, and it lasted throughout the entire year-long study." There is no medical treatment that can even come close to having such a high effectiveness rate.

At the beginning of the program participants ate a detoxifying type of diet for one week. It consisted of herbal teas, vegetable broths, and carrot, beet, celery, and potato juices. For the next three to five months they ate a vegan diet—no animal products at all, which means no meat, fish, milk, poultry, and eggs. They also avoided gluten, refined sugar, citrus fruits, strong spices, and preservatives. Next they added foods back one by one. If they observed a flare-up within a twenty-four- to forty-eight-hour period after eating the food, they rejected that food for one week and then reintroduced it again. If after the second attempt to include it in their diet they saw another flare-up of symptoms, they avoided the food for the remainder of the study.

Dr. Kjeldsen-Kragh concluded that approximately 70 percent of people saw improvement in inflammation and pain because they avoided the wrong kinds of fats, namely from meat, which is well known to worsen the inflammation process. Others saw improvements because they excluded foods to which they were sensitive or allergic.

In my clinical experience as a nutritionist and doctor of natural medicine for twenty-five years, I believe that most arthritics eat far more meat and inflammatory fats in their diet than their body can handle.

Plant Power

Many different fruits, vegetables, nuts, and seeds contain compounds that help heal arthritis. Most colorful fruits and vegetables contain healing phytochemicals (plant chemicals) that reduce inflammation. Specific food compounds known as flavonoids (also called vitamin P) help with healing and injuries as well by increasing the absorption of vitamin C and have healing properties themselves. For example, flavonoids improve blood vessel health, and blood vessels feed the joints with oxygen-rich blood. Flavonoids also have anti-inflammatory properties due to their antioxidant properties and their ability to act against histamines and other substances linked with inflammation, namely prostaglandins and leukotrienes. Many nuts and seeds contain healthy fats and protein as well as vitamins and minerals. Some of the best healing remedies to overcome inflammation also taste fabulous (I can't say that about any prescription medications). Plus, foods won't cause the nasty side effects common to most pain medications. Here are some of the best plant-powered foods that act as medicine in the body:

THE BENEFITS OF CHERRIES AND BERRIES

Although many people opt for aspirin as their first course of action when they incur an injury, Muraleedharan Nair, PhD and professor of natural products and chemistry at Michigan State University, found that tart cherry extract is ten times more effective than aspirin at alleviating inflammation. Only two tablespoons of the concentrated juice, which is found in many health food stores, needs to be taken daily for effective results. Later she found that sweet cherries, blackberries, raspberries, and strawberries have similar effects. Of course, eating a half cup or more of cherries or berries on a regular basis can provide pain and inflammation relief.

Blueberries are also excellent anti-inflammatory agents. They increase the amounts of compounds called heat-shock proteins, which decrease as people age, thereby causing inflammation and damage. By eating blueberries regularly, research shows that these heat-shock proteins stop declining; inflammation lessens, and pain decreases, not to mention they just taste fabulous.

When my mother quit smoking she started eating frozen blueberries as her treat instead of smoking cigarettes. Later she told me about this newly found habit. Frozen blueberries taste like blueberry sorbet and make a delicious anti-arthritis treat instead of unhealthy sweets.

THE CELERY SENSATION

Consider celery: James Duke, PhD, author of *The Green Pharmacy*, found more than twenty anti-inflammatory compounds in celery and celery seeds, including a substance called apigenin, which is powerful in its anti-inflammatory action. Incidentally Hildegard von Bingen, writer, scientist, musician, nun, and visionary, wrote about celery's anti-inflammatory properties over nine hundred years ago. If you're not sure how to use celery seeds, add them to soups, stews, or as a salt substitute in many recipes. Celery seed bread made with gluten-free bread is one of my favorite foods and makes an excellent side dish or appetizer of in place of garlic bread. Simply brush olive oil on gluten-free whole-grain bread and sprinkle with celery seeds, bake in a 300 degree Fahrenheit oven until golden brown, and serve immediately.

PINEAPPLE POWER

Pineapple is one of the notable anti-arthritic foods, as it contains the powerful anti-inflammatory enzyme known as bromelain, which we'll discuss further in chapter 4. But for now include small amounts of fresh—not canned—pineapple; only the fresh pineapple contains the beneficial enzymes.

OUTRUN PAIN WITH HOT PEPPERS

I know this sounds crazy. After all, how can hot peppers outrun pain? But research shows that capsaicin, the ingredient that gives hot peppers their fireworks, alleviates pain by traveling the same pathways as pain to the brain. It's similar to a race where the fastest runner crosses the finish line first; in this race capsaicin travels much faster than the fastest pain signals, meaning it will always win. And that's great news for you: whether you're suffering from muscle pain, joint pain, or even nerve pain, capsaicin works.

Dull pain travels at one-half to two miles per second. Sharp or burning pain travels at five to thirty miles per second. Capsaicin follows the same pathway through the nerves in the spinal cord to the brain, at between thirty-five to seventy-five miles per second. Not even Usain Bolt, the fastest man in the world, can compete with that kind of speed. That's why ointments or oils that contain capsaicin and are applied to sore muscles or joints work—that hot sensation you feel on the skin literally outruns most forms of pain to get to your brain, which blocks the perception of other pain so that its effects are muted, if not stopped completely!

You can also benefit from eating spicy food made with chili peppers or by taking supplements containing capsaicin. Ironically, cayenne pepper turns *down* the heat on inflammation due to its powerful anti-inflammatory compound, capsaicin.

ORANGE, RED, AND GREEN POWER

As you can see, fighting arthritis is not all about eliminating foods you may have enjoyed; delicious and nutritious food can also be the best medicine. Some fruits and vegetables contain special plant compounds, phytonutrients, known as astaxanthin, which can help with arthritis. Astaxanthin is particularly found in many orange, red, and green fruits and vegetables, including carrots, squashes, pumpkin, leafy greens, broccoli, pomegranates, and beets. Supplementary astaxanthin may also help with arthritis. We'll discuss more about the anti-inflammatory and antipain properties of this nutritional supplement in chapter 5.

POMEGRANATE POWER

Eat pomegranates to reduce inflammation and joint pain. Researchers at Case Western Reserve University in Cleveland, Ohio, studied the effects of pomegranate fruit extract on classical markers of inflammation and cartilage degradation in arthritic joints. These markers, referred to as matrix metallo-proteinases (MMPs), are a family of enzymes that facilitate a wide variety of functions in the body; however, the uncontrolled regulation and enhanced expression of MMPs is linked with the development of arthritis.[13]

Additionally, pomegranates fight harmful bacteria. Researchers in South Africa evaluated the antibacterial, antioxidant, and other activities of extracts from peels of seven commercially grown pomegranate cultivars. They determined that peel extracts showed strong broad-spectrum activity against a variety of different bacteria known as gram-positive and gram-negative bacteria and concluded that pomegranate fruit peel has potential as a safe and natural antimicrobial agent.[14]

Enjoy pomegranate seeds fresh from the fruit by cutting it in half and pulling them from the off-white flesh of the fruit. The seeds are delicious on their own or added to your favorite brown rice or quinoa dish for an explosion of taste or on top of Greek yogurt. You can also wash the peel of organic pomegranate fruits and brew a tea with it.

GREEN REIGNS SUPREME

In addition to containing the antipain compound known as astaxanthin, dark green veggies like kale and spinach contain high amounts of minerals like calcium and magnesium. Both minerals help alleviate inflammation and support healthy joints, muscles, and ligaments. Calcium and magnesium are both needed in sufficient quantities to regulate pain signals in the brain and nervous system. Additionally, magnesium helps reduce the pain and tightness of the muscle tension involved in fibromyalgia.

MAX FLAX FOR MAX HEALING

Flaxseeds and the oil derived from these miniature healers are high in natural omega 3 that convert into hormone-like substances in the body to reduce inflammatory substances. We discussed flax earlier, but it bears inclusion here among the best plant-based foods to add to your diet. Add ground flax seeds to smoothies or atop pancakes, gluten-free French toast, oatmeal, and many other foods. To keep the omega 3 fatty acids intact and capable of quelling inflammation in your body, do not heat them.

GINGER POWER

Dr. Krishna C. Srivastava at Odense University in Denmark found that ginger was superior to nonsteroidal anti-inflammatory drugs (NSAIDs) like Tylenol or Advil at alleviating inflammation. We'll discuss ginger in greater detail in chapter 5.

CURRY CAPACITY

If you've ever eaten an Indian curry, you're probably familiar with turmeric. It is the yellowish spice commonly used in Indian cuisine. While it adds delicious flavor to your meals, it also offers many benefits to your health. Curcumin, the primary active ingredient in turmeric, has antipain and anti-inflammatory properties. Research shows that the Indian spice frequently used in curries suppresses pain and inflammation through a similar mechanism as drugs like COX-1 and COX-2 inhibitors, but without the harmful side effects. Additionally, new research indicates that ingesting 1200mg of curcumin, the main therapeutic constituent of the spice turmeric, had the same effect as taking 300mg of the potent anti-inflammatory drug phenylbutazone.

WALNUT WELLNESS

Like flaxseeds, raw, unsalted walnuts contain plentiful amounts of omega 3 fatty acids that decrease pain and inflammation. Raw walnuts make a delicious snack, and walnut oil adds a delightful nutty flavor to salad dressings and meals cooked with it.

SUMMARY OF THE BEST ANTI-ARTHRITIS FOODS TO EAT

There are many great foods to enjoy on an arthritis-recovery plan. The following are among the best anti-arthritis foods to eat.

- celery and celery seeds
- fatty fish (like salmon, mackerel, herring, sardines, and tuna; see the section on fish and gout on page 65 if you suffer from gout)
- flax oil, walnut oil, hemp oil, or extra-virgin olive oil
- fresh raw nuts, especially walnuts and almonds (including almond milk and walnut oil)
- fresh, raw vegetable and fruit juices
- fruits and vegetables (enjoy a wide variety of cooked and raw fruits and vegetables; try to eat as many raw fruits and vegetables as possible to boost the healing enzymes in your body)

- **gluten-free whole grains and legumes like brown rice, millet, quinoa, and wild rice**

- **leafy greens like spinach, dandelion greens, and kale**

- **orange, red, and green fruits and vegetables**

- **raw apples, pineapple, and berries like blueberries, blackberries, pomegranates, raspberries, strawberries, and cherries**

- **spices like turmeric, garlic, cloves, onions, ginger, celery seeds, turmeric, chili peppers, licorice (the herb), and peppermint**

Spice Up Your Life

Whenever someone tells me that healthy food is bland and boring, I remind them that there is a world of spices out there to give any meal a flavor boost, from salads to fish to desserts. Not only do spices create new twists on old food favorites, they also often contain incredible pain-busting and inflammation-reducing compounds. The following are the top ten anti-inflammatory and antipain spices.

1. turmeric
2. celery seeds
3. garlic
4. ginger
5. cloves
6. chili peppers (capsaicin)
7. licorice (not the stuff you find at movie theaters and variety stores; use only real licorice, the herb)
8. peppermint
9. paprika
10. onion

Diet helps regulate the body's inflammatory agents, and avoiding certain types of food can elicit a powerful anti-inflammatory response in the body. By eating a vegetarian or predominantly vegetarian diet (fish can be included in the diet if you prefer, but be careful which kinds and how much you include if you suffer from gout) high in critical nutrients found in spices like ginger, garlic, and onions; loaded with berries and cherries; and plenty of phytonutrient-rich fruits and vegetables, you will experience tremendous joint and overall bodily healing.

Choose Organic as Much as Possible

In study after study research from independent organizations consistently shows organic food is higher in nutrients than industrially farmed foods. Research shows that organic produce is higher in vitamin C, antioxidants, and the minerals calcium, iron, chromium, and magnesium.

Nonorganic foods contain neurotoxins, which are damaging to brain and nerve cells. A commonly used class of pesticides called organophosphates was originally developed as a toxic nerve agent during World War I. When there was no longer a need for them in warfare, industry adapted them to kill pests on foods. Many pesticides are still considered neurotoxins that impact the brain and nervous system, which is responsible for controlling pain signals. Why take a chance that toxic pesticides interfere with the smooth functioning of this important system?

They are real food, not pesticide factories, which may sound outlandish, but bear with me. Genetically modified (GM) corn is well known for its inflammation-causing properties. Additionally, most GM corn contains the toxic pesticide glyphosate in every cell. The main ingredient in this pesticide, glyphosate, was recently declared a carcinogen by the World Health Organization. Although I'm not aware of any studies exploring other possible links besides glyphosate's inflammatory effects, between arthritis and glyphosate, it's best to avoid GM foods as much as possible, and the best way to do that is to eat more organic foods.

Some nonorganic food—such as fruits and vegetables, including avocadoes, bananas and tomatoes—is exposed to gas-ripening. Ethylene gas is sprayed on fruit that was picked prematurely, before it was sufficiently ripe, to encourage ripening after transportation. While fruits and vegetables naturally emit ethylene gas during ripening, it is unclear whether there are differences between the natural off-gassing process and being spray-gassed with ethylene, sourced from ethanol, in a warehouse. Ethanol is usually derived from corn, which is largely genetically-modified. Most genetically-modified organisms (GMOs) have been linked to inflammation in humans, and are best avoided.

As we discussed earlier, choosing organic meat decreases your exposure to antibiotics, synthetic hormones, and drugs that find their way into the animals and, ultimately, into you. These substances can throw off the delicate microbial balance in our intestines or our hormonal balance. As we'll discuss later in this book, microbial balance in the gut is imperative to a healthy immune system and even healthy joints.

Organic food is tried and tested. By some estimates GM food makes up 75 to 80 percent of the average person's food consumption. Genetic modification of food is still experimental, and as I mentioned earlier, has been linked to inflammation. Additionally, it has been linked to cancer, birth defects, and other serious health issues. Plus, most organic food simply tastes better than the pesticide-grown counterparts. The taste difference surprises most people.

Your Watery Inner World

We constantly hear about the importance of drinking enough water. On the flip side, there has been a growing trend in the media lately, telling us that the recommended eight cups of water daily is a myth, which is technically accurate, but not the whole story. Whether you need eight cups of water daily or four or ten, most people are not getting the message that whatever their particular water needs are, they aren't meeting them.

And even dieticians, nutritionists, and medical professionals are contributing to the problem by informing people that they get enough water in their diet in the form of fruits and vegetables. That might be true for some people, but after assessing the diets of countless people, I assure you that isn't the case for most people. Plus, have you ever noticed that when you throw vegetables in a pan and turn on the heat you see liquid in the pan soon afterward and then shortly after that you'll see steam rising from them? That's because you're literally cooking the water out of the vegetables.

Researchers estimate that half of the world's population is chronically dehydrated. And in America, that level is even higher—at 75 percent of the population. In my experience most people who are experiencing pain or illness are chronically dehydrated. Plain and simple.

More than two-thirds of your body weight is water. Every cell and organ requires adequate water to function properly. Without adequate water your body's biochemical and electrical functions begin to break down. And what is one of the primary electrical functions in your body? Pain signals that travel via electrical signals through the nervous system and brain. The list of reasons your body needs water is as plentiful as the functions in your body, so due to space limitations, here are ten good reasons to drink more water.

1. Water lubricates our joints and helps reduce joint pain.
2. Your blood is over 80 percent water and needs water to make healthy new oxygen-rich blood cells that support healthy joints and tissues.
3. Your bones are over 50 percent water and, you guessed it, need water to make healthy new bone cells.
4. Drinking more water actually helps lessen pain in your body by getting your lymphatic system moving. The

lymphatic system is a network of nodes, tubes, and vessels that move waste out of your tissues, and it requires water to function properly.

5. Water helps eliminate wastes and toxins from your body via the kidneys and intestines.
6. Water regulates metabolism, so if you're overweight, chances are you may need more water.
7. Water balances body temperature.
8. Water helps ensure adequate electrical functioning so our brain and nervous system functions properly.
9. Every cell and organ requires adequate water to function properly.
10. Water alleviates dehydration—and we already established that most people, particularly those suffering from pain, are chronically dehydrated.

So one of the quickest and easiest ways to improve your health and the health of your joints is to start drinking more pure water every day. Be sure to drink water on an empty stomach, or you'll simply be diluting your digestive enzymes and making your digestion less effective. In wealthy, developed nations with plentiful access to water, we really have no excuses for not drinking enough. Of course, you can still drink enough water with meals to take any supplements or medications that need to be taken with food.

A SENSITIVE MATTER

Many arthritics are suffering from food sensitivities that aggravate their condition. Some of the main food sensitivities arthritics experience include corn, wheat, rye bread, pork and bacon, eggs, coffee, dairy products, chocolate, oranges, beef, and eggs.

Dr. D. N. Golding, a rheumatologist at Princess Alexandra Hospital in Harlow, Essex, England, discovered something that he calls "allergic synovitis," which is inflammation of the syno-vial membrane that secretes fluid in the joint cavities to keep the joints lubricated and moving smoothly. Joint pain typically follows inflammation, and the people most often struck with inflammation and pain are those with allergies, especially those who experience other allergic types of symptoms such as rashes, hives, and hay fever. Dr. Golding cites dairy products, includ-ing cheese, and eggs as the most common culprits of "allergic synovitis."

Food sensitivities play a surprisingly important role in arthri-tis. Many arthritics discover that common breakfast foods like bacon, eggs, coffee, and dairy products aggravate their condi-tion. Other common food sensitivities linked to arthritis include wheat and gluten, rye bread, corn, beef, chocolate, and oranges.

Keep in mind that it can take up to forty-eight hours for these types of sensitive reactions to manifest. In that time, if you've eaten another common allergen, it is unlikely you'll be able to link the joint pain, swelling, and other arthritic reactions to the foods you're eating. Instead, you will have ongoing, pain-ful symptoms of arthritis and will not even realize the connec-tion between your symptoms and the foods you are eating. As a result, it is best to eliminate the common allergens for at least a couple of weeks and then introduce one food item that causes allergic reactions back into your diet. Wait for forty-eight hours to see whether you have any reaction to the food or aggravation of your arthritis symptoms.

In addition to the common allergens mentioned earlier, tomatoes, bell peppers, and potatoes can sometimes aggravate arthritis. Although tomatoes and bell peppers contain about twenty anti-inflammatory substances each, some arthritics may be sensitive to this group of foods known as nightshades. This group includes tomatoes and bell peppers as well as white pota-toes (not sweet potatoes), so it's best to avoid them at first and then introduce them into your diet to see whether you have any reaction. Further, some of the heightened sensitivity to foods many people are experiencing may actually be to pesticides or GMOs, so you may find that by eating more organic foods, you reduce your likelihood of experiencing food sensitivities.

The simple act of eating is a significant factor in your health or lack of health, depending on your food choices. If you're like most people, you probably don't realize just how important this daily act can be. The foods you choose can either aggravate your arthritis symptoms or reverse the inflammation and pain you experience. Although it may be hard to imagine that the food you eat can play a bigger role in how you feel than the medications you take, it's true. And once you've experienced the healing power of delicious, natural foods, you'll never want to go back to your old eating habits.

Special Food Considerations for Gout

In the case of gout, a form of arthritis primarily affecting the big toe, there are many specific foods that can aggravate the condition, namely foods that contain purines. Your body produces uric acid to help break down these purine-rich foods. Over time this uric acid can become deposited in the joints. The big toe seems most vulnerable to uric acid crystals. The following are some of the foods with the highest levels of purines, which means they are among those most likely to aggravate gout:

- organ meats such as liver and giblets
- red meat, including beef, bison, lamb, and pork
- fish and seafood, especially anchovies, herring, and mackerel
- alcohol, especially beer
- foods and drinks sweetened with high-fructose corn syrup, including many soft drinks and sweetened juices; juices that are made from 100 percent fruit are not nearly as problematic

SIMPLE SWITCHES TO ARTHRITIS-PROOF YOUR LIFE

The old adage "you are what you eat" is easily tested on most arthritis sufferers. If you start your day with bacon and eggs, coffee and milk, and a cheese Danish, lunch on pizza and cola, and dine on steak and French fries, your joints will hurt. Your body is screaming at you, "Enough!" If you made an honest attempt to replace one of these items every week, you will experience a significant reduction in pain and inflammation. It may take some time for your body to start healing from the inflammation these foods can cause or aggravate. Here are some suggestions:

- Replace the bacon and eggs with unsweetened oatmeal or a fruit and berry plate.
- Replace the coffee and milk with green tea (hot or cold) and lemon.
- Replace the cheese Danish with whole-grain gluten-free toast and raw, organic almond butter.
- Replace pizza with a mixed green salad (homemade dressing with cold-pressed flax, walnut, or olive oil) with raw, unsalted walnuts and an avocado, lettuce, and cucumber sandwich on 100 percent whole-grain gluten-free bread.
- Replace the cola with water, lemon water, ginger tea (hot or cold), or a fresh-squeezed vegetable juice.
- Replace the steak with wild salmon or grilled Portobello mushrooms.
- Replace the French fries with baked sweet potato fries tossed in a small amount of olive or walnut oil. Alternatively, choose a mixed green salad, lightly grilled squash or curried vegetables, tossed with a walnut oil and lemon juice vinaigrette.
- Replace the fast food snacks with berries (fresh or frozen), raw fruit, and carrot and celery sticks with almond butter.

3

Addressing an Almost Unknown Cause of Arthritis

ORTHOMOLECULAR MEDICINE IS A branch of medicine that was first conceptualized by double–Nobel laureate Linus Pauling in 1968. It involves correcting molecular imbalances in the body on the basis of individual biochemistry using critical nutrients.[1] Dr. Pauling discovered that many of his patients showed mental signs of vitamin deficiencies long before physical symptoms appeared. He proceeded to treat his patients with specific nutrients and achieved a reversal of the symptoms of mental illnesses, including schizophrenia, and published his first paper, "Orthomolecular Psychiatry," on his clinical results in the medical journal *Science*.[2] Over his lifetime he proceeded to test his theories on many other health conditions with impressive results, which he published in numerous scientific papers and books.

Since then the field of orthomolecular medicine, or orthomo-lecular nutrition as it is also called, has developed into a complete system of medicine many doctors and nutritionists around the world practice and has been used to effectively treat many serious health conditions, including osteoarthritis and rheumatoid arthritis. There is an association known as the International Society of Orthomolecular Medicine (ISOM), with chapters in many countries around the world.

Although many health practitioners incorporate vitamin, mineral, and other nutritional supplements into the management of their patients' health conditions, the field of orthomolecular medicine is different in that it involves identifying underlying deficiencies that may be involved in a person's disease or disorder and then determining the right dose, at the right time, and taken at the right frequency to obtain maximum results. This approach has proven itself immensely effective in the treatment of many conditions, including arthritis.

Orthomolecular medical research shows how correcting two critical nutritional deficiencies can stop the progression of arthritis in its tracks in most cases and even reverse some cases of arthritis. Yet most doctors and nutritionists have not even heard of this groundbreaking research. I'll also share insights into how you can benefit from this exciting and potentially life-changing research.

Before diving into the specific nutrients, dosages, and frequencies, let's explore the history of how the nutritional deficiencies involved in arthritis were discovered. I think you'll find it fascinating, and the story may leave you with some questions as to why these amazing marvels of medicine have not been further espoused.

A BRIEF ORTHOMOLECULAR HISTORY OF ARTHRITIS

In 1943 a physician named Dr. William Kaufman wrote and published a book entitled *The Common Form of Niacin Amide*

Deficiency Disease: Aniacinamidosis. He had discovered that many people seemed to be suffering from some common symptoms that he recognized as manifestations of vitamin B3, or niacin, deficiency. Some of these symptoms included:

- depression, or "inappropriate" moods, as he described them
- difficulty in comprehension
- distractability
- impaired memory
- impatience
- insomnia
- irritability
- lack of initiative
- mental fog
- paranoid personality
- poor balance
- tension
- unwarranted anxiety and fear

He believed these symptoms were the early stages of a condition known as pellagra, a deficiency of vitamin B3 (niacin) that is characterized by gastrointestinal disorders, dermatitis, premature aging, neurological conditions, and reduced immunity to infectious diseases.

Dr. Kaufman devoted a chapter in his book to arthritis, in which he theorized that subclinical pellagra may lead to impaired muscle strength and endurance as well as the impairment of joint mobility and tenderness of the cartilage and membranes surrounding bones. He stated, "In persons suffering from aniacinamidosis, there occurs a progressive clinical pattern that, in its final stages, is diagnosed arthritis." Sadly, although he made this discovery almost seventy-three years ago, it is as groundbreaking today as it was in 1943.

Dr. Kaufman proceeded to give his patients 1000mg of niacinamide (a type of niacin that does not cause what is known as "niacin flush," in which people experience a heat sensation throughout their body) daily and observed vast improvements in their arthritic conditions.

Around the same time vitamin B3 began to be added to flour— what we now know as "enriched flour." Dr. Kaufman observed that many people no longer had the subclinical symptoms of niacin deficiency mentioned above but still had marked symptoms of arthritis. He theorized that arthritis was a severe niacin deficiency and began giving his patients higher doses of the vitamin—up to 4000mg daily in divided doses. He had impressive results and published a second book, this time devoted to the subject of arthritis, entitled, *The Common Form of Joint Dysfunction*. He found that, for some unknown reason, some people were vulnerable to the effects of a vitamin B3 deficiency that could not be resolved with diet alone. In other words, these people needed higher doses of vitamin B3, or niacin, than could be obtained through foods in their diet. Dr. Kaufman drew these conclusions from his 455 arthritic patients he treated and whose responses to vitamin B3 he studied over the course of two years.

Obviously not every arthritis sufferer is severely deficient in this vitamin or is deficient in it at all, but according to Dr. Kaufman's research, many people are needlessly suffering from a disease that is not recognized as a serious vitamin deficiency. Although his research took place decades ago and has been largely forgotten, overlooked, or suppressed, many orthomolecular nutritionists or orthomolecular medicine practitioners can attest that they have had similar impressive results by prescribing high doses of vitamin B3 for their arthritic patients.

Although many people—doctors included—used to believe that vitamins didn't have much of an effect on health, that idea has long been considered a medical myth. The reality is that nutrients impact every part of your body. Vitamins, minerals,

phytonutrients (special plant nutrients), amino acids (the building blocks of protein), essential fats, carbs, enzymes (which we'll
discuss in the next chapter), and other nutrients are needed in
sufficient amounts to make healthy cells, tissues, glands, bones,
joints, organs, and organ systems. After years of extensive
research we now know that vitamins, to use just one example,
by definition are required for health. After all, the Oxford Dic-
tionary definition of a *vitamin* is "any of a group of organic compounds which are essential for normal growth and nutrition and
are required in small quantities in the diet because they cannot
be synthesized by the body."[3]

Every cell in your body needs particular vitamins to work
properly. Without adequate vitamins, cellular functions begin
to break down until there are potentially serious flaws in their
workings. If this happens, the cells may even die off prematurely
as the body tries to protect itself against possible damage. Alternatively, defective cells form the basis of tissues in the body,
which can then result in disease or impaired function.

If even a single vitamin is deficient in the body, the results
can be disastrous to our health. And by now you're probably
beginning to understand that some people simply have higher
needs for specific vitamins than others. The reality is that
everyone is biochemically unique, and although we all need
vitamins, minerals, and other nutrients for our survival and
optimal health, we need them in different quantities than the
recommended dietary intakes (RDIs) that government bodies put forth. In the case of people vulnerable to arthritis, it
seems that a large proportion have a vitamin B3 deficiency
that cannot be restored through food alone. So no matter how
many niacin-rich foods are eaten, the amount is unlikely to
be sufficient.

Our current lifestyle can also deplete already insufficient
dietary intakes of niacin. Stress, alcohol consumption, the use of
some prescription drugs, poor digestion or nutrient absorption

can also lead to deficiencies in this important nutrient. Niacin is only one of a whole complex of vitamins known as *B vitamins*.

There are many B vitamins, including thiamin (B1), riboflavin (B2), niacin (B3), pantothenic acid (B5), pyridoxine (B6), folate (B9), cobalamin (B12), B13 (orotic acid), B15 (pangamic acid), and B17 (amygdalin, or laetrile if it is synthetic). Additionally, there are other nutrients that comprise the B vitamin complex, including choline, inositol, biotin, and PABA. B complex vitamins are needed for many bodily functions, including manufacturing hormones, supplying energy to cells, immune system health, pain reduction, and proper pain signaling, to name a few.

Although most B vitamins can be found in foods like eggs, fish, legumes, whole grains, nuts, brown rice, root vegetables, pumpkin seeds, citrus fruits, strawberries, cantaloupe, kale, green vegetables, and most beans, for many people suffering from arthritis, they are found in insufficient amounts. In addition to adding more of these foods to your diet, it is wise to take a B complex supplement as well. Alternatively, be sure that your high-quality multivitamin contains at least 50 to 100mg of adequate B vitamins. Note that some of the B vitamins, such as folate and cobalamin, are measured in micrograms; B complex or multivitamins should contain 50 to 100 micrograms of these specific vitamins. Although the B-complex vitamins they work best when taken together, it is also imperative for anyone with arthritis to address a possible underlying niacin dependency or deficiency by taking extra niacin in the form of niacin, nicotinic acid, or niacinamide. Without addressing a niacin deficiency or dependency, people suffering from arthritis may simply have minimal or short-lived symptom improvement without ever significantly affecting the condition.

Although niacin and nicotinic acid are excellent forms of vitamin B3, they can cause what is known as a *niacin flush*, a sensation that involves heat and tingling throughout the body. The synthetic form of the vitamin, known as niacinamide, has many of the same beneficial effects as the natural forms but does not cause this flush, making it a superior choice for anyone wishing to avoid an uncomfortable flushing effect. A niacin flush is not dangerous but can be uncomfortable for some people.

Niacinamide supplementation seems to improve joint mobility, pain, and swelling.[4] Start with 500mg of niacinamide taken three times daily, and gradually increase to 3000mg. If after one month you still haven't seen noticeable results in your arthritis symptoms, increase the amount of niacin to 4000mg. This supplementation is best followed by a physician or an orthomolecular nutritionist during this time, as many arthritics taking high doses of this nutrient may be able to reduce their dosages of pain-killing drugs.

THE NUTRIENT-HOMOCYSTEINE CONNECTION

A growing body of research links a chemical produced in the body to an increasing number of serious health conditions, including rheumatoid arthritis and heart disease. Fortunately new research also shows that high levels of this damaging chemical can often be reversed with nutritional supplementation.

What Is Homocysteine?

Homocysteine is a type of protein produced by the body and found in the blood. It is ideally found in low levels. Produced from an amino acid called methionine, which is found in protein foods in the diet, the body normally turns homocysteine into beneficial substances like glutathione or S-adenosylmethionine (SAMe). The former is heavily involved in the detoxification of harmful substances and the latter is involved in virtually every biochemical process in the body, including the maintenance of healthy joints.[5]

Risk Factors for High Homocysteine Levels

There are numerous risk factors that can result in high levels of homocysteine, including:[6]

- genetics: a family history of heart disease, strokes, cancer, Alzheimer's disease, schizophrenia, diabetes, or the MTHFR enzyme gene mutation that can increase the amount of homocysteine in the body
- less than 900mcg/day of folate
- increasing age
- male gender
- deficiency in estrogen
- excessive alcohol, coffee, or tea intake
- smoking
- lack of exercise
- hostility and repressed anger
- inflammatory bowel disease like celiac, Crohn's, or ulcerative colitis
- *H. pylori*–generated ulcers
- pregnancy
- strict veganism or vegetarianism
- high-fat diet with excessive red meat; high-fat dairy intake
- high salt intake

Concerns About Homocysteine

Homocysteine damages the joints, arteries, brain, and genetic material (DNA) and can increase the risk for over fifty diseases,[7] including rheumatoid arthritis,[8] Alzheimer's disease, cancer, depression, diabetes, heart attack, stroke, and rheumatoid arthritis.

Your doctor can request blood tests to determine whether your levels of homocysteine are high. Fortunately, even if they are high, homocysteine levels frequently drop in response to a low-sugar, plant-based diet high in nutrients like the ones outlined in the last chapter.

Dietary Approaches for Reducing Homocysteine Levels

It is possible to reduce homocysteine levels by following a healthy diet comprising the following suggestions:

- Eat less fatty meat and more fish and plant-based protein.
- Eat green vegetables and leafy greens, which are high in B complex vitamins, including vitamin B6, B12, and folate.
- Eat gluten-free whole grains because they are also high in B complex vitamins.
- Have a clove of garlic a day.
- Don't add salt to your food.
- Cut back on tea and coffee.
- Limit your alcohol.
- Reduce your stress levels as much as possible.
- Stop smoking.
- Supplement with a high-strength multivitamin every day.

If you are following the eating program outlined in the last chapter, you'll notice that you are well on your way to following the dietary approach necessary to reduce homocysteine levels.

Nutritional Supplements

Supplementing your diet with B complex vitamins can be helpful because you need them to activate the enzymes that turn harmful homocysteine into beneficial nutrients like glutathione or SAMe. Without adequate amounts of these vitamins, homocysteine will not be converted to these beneficial substances, resulting in dangerously high levels of homocysteine and potentially low levels of the beneficial glutathione and SAMe. Research shows that supplementary folic acid and vitamin B12 can make the deficient enzyme work more effectively.[9]

In a study published in the *Scandinavian Journal of Rheumatology*, researchers found that supplementation with vitamins B6, folate (B9), and B12 (cobalamin) could significantly reduce homocysteine levels in people suffering from rheumatoid arthritis.[10] Reducing homocysteine levels results in a significant reduction in inflammation as well.

Take a B complex vitamin supplement containing 100mg of the B vitamins daily. Some of the B vitamins such as folate and B12 are measured in micrograms; the supplement should contain 100 micrograms of these B vitamins. It is fine to take the B complex vitamin supplement in addition to extra niacin and folate mentioned above. For example, if your B complex contains 100 micrograms of folate and you're trying to take 400 micrograms of folate daily, simply subtract 100 from 400 to obtain the amount of folate you can take on its own (300 micrograms).

How to Find Out If Your Homocysteine Levels Are High

High homocysteine can be identified through urine tests that show homocystinuria, the increased presence of homocystine, which is a double molecule of homocysteine.[11] The average level is 10 units (millimole/liter); ideal readings are below 6 units.

FOLIC ACID

In addition to its role in reducing homocysteine in the body, research has established a link between a folic acid deficiency and rheumatoid arthritis. You may recall that folic acid, or folate as it is also known, was one of the top-prescribed medications for arthritis, making folic acid a supplement of choice among natural health professionals and medical doctors alike.

As early as 1964 the *British Medical Journal* reported on a link between a folic acid deficiency and rheumatoid arthritis.[12] In the study researchers found that participants with rheumatoid arthritis had significantly lower levels of folic acid than those acting as controls.

Folic acid reduces homocysteine levels, boosts healthy cell growth needed for joint and tissue repair, aids in the formation of DNA at the cellular level, and helps protect DNA from damage linked to disease.[13]

Fortunately folic acid is affordable and readily available. Start with 400 *micro*grams of folic acid, or folate, daily unless you are pregnant or breastfeeding, in which case you should take 600 micrograms during pregnancy and 500 micrograms if you are breastfeeding. As with most nutrients, continue taking folic acid daily for at least three months to see results.

Folic acid, like other B complex vitamins, is water soluble, which means you'll need to take it every day because it won't be stored in your body. There is little to no risk in taking excess amounts of water-soluble vitamins, as the body simply eliminates any excess in the urine. But many arthritics will absorb most of the B vitamins they take because they tend to be deficient in these nutrients. Some people wrongly assume that because their urine gets brighter yellow while taking B vitamins, they are paying for expensive urine, but that's just not the case. While vitamin B6 does change the color of the urine, it helps to protect the urinary tract from damage. I've also come across research that shows B complex vitamins in the urine actually help protect against cancer of the urinary tract, so consider it a protective measure.

Folic acid can be found in most green leafy vegetables such as spinach and kale as well as most fruits, especially citrus fruits, dried peas and beans, and whole grains. Although it is valuable to eat a diet rich in folic acid–containing foods, most arthritics need to supplement with this nutrient to obtain sufficient quantities in their diet.

VITAMIN *B12*

Like folic acid, vitamin B12 helps heal arthritis. Vitamin B12 is actually a number of nutrients known as cobalamins. It comes in

different forms, including methylcobalamin and hydroxycobala-
min, both of which are good forms with which to supplement.

Like folic acid, vitamin B12 helps form the genetic material
in the cells. It is also used to create energy at the cellular level, a
key role vital to every cellular function in the body, as every biochemical reaction in the body needs sufficient energy. Vitamin
B12 also helps convert folic acid into its active form in the body
so it can be properly used.[14] Because they work so well together,
vitamin B12 and folic acid are best taken together.

They usually come in a B complex supplement, but you'll usually need more than what a typical B complex supplement offers.
As a result, I recommend taking a B complex supplement every
day, as suggested above. Additionally, I suggest extra folic acid
and B12, which sometimes come together in a single supplement but more are available as individual nutrients. In addition
to the amount of folic acid recommended above, be sure to take
1000 *micro*grams of B12. If you're getting 100 micrograms in a
B complex vitamin and an extra 1,000 micrograms of B12 in
a separate supplement, totaling 1,100 micrograms, that's fine.
Your body will use most if not all of it and will simply excrete
any excess in the urine. In the case of arthritis, plenty of energy
is needed at the cellular level for adequate healing, so you'll
likely absorb plentiful amounts of this nutrient.

Most people notice an increase in energy while taking B complex supplements in general and B12 in particular. This is typically
a welcome side effect, but you may want to take your B vitamins
in the morning or early afternoon before 3 p.m. to avoid any inter-
ference with your sleep. Vitamin B12 is also found in salmon, eggs,
clams, sprouts, and the blue-green algae powder spirulina, but
most arthritics need to supplement with this nutrient to obtain
sufficient amounts in their daily diet. Addressing these nutritional
deficiencies can go a long way toward healing arthritic symptoms
and halting the worsening of the disease.

4

Enzymes: Miracle Warriors
Against Arthritis

I N SOME CULTURES LANGUAGE is more than a way of communicating; it is an expression of the most important components of daily life. For example, every symbol in the ancient Norse alphabet represents a particular aspect of primeval life. A particular S-like letter resembled a lightning strike and represented both the sun's energy and the spark of energy they recognized as existing within all living beings. They treated both the sun's energy and the human life force energy as sacred.

Most of us are aware that we are more than a collection of bones, joints, muscles, cells, and other physical structures. Although these body parts are obviously important, as are the many biochemical processes that occur within our bodies, we are not simply the sum of these parts and processes; indeed, there is a spark that initiates and organizes processes within our body to keep us alive, functioning, and healthy. From a biochemical viewpoint that spark comes in the form of enzymes, specialized forms of proteins that ensure every cellular and biochemical process can occur in the body. Enzymes act as catalysts to initiate, activate, or expedite virtually every process in the body. Unlike other types of protein molecules, enzymes are biologically active. In other words, they contain life-force energy that act as sparks to awaken and incite the various processes in the body. We could not live without enzymes.

Extensive research by one of the earliest enzymologists, Dr. Edward Howell, revealed that enzyme shortages are commonly seen in people suffering from chronic diseases, including arthritis, allergies, premature aging, cancer, heart disease, skin conditions, and obesity.

Enzymes are used in vast quantities in our bodies to quell inflammation, promote joint (and other types of) healing, regenerate tissues, all of which are essential processes involved in arthritis. So it should come as no surprise that illness and injury may deplete our body's ability to manufacture sufficient enzymes to ensure these processes occur smoothly and to aid joint healing. There are three main types of enzymes: metabolic, digestive, and food enzymes.

Metabolic enzymes. The body makes metabolic enzymes to properly run all of its biochemical processes, from moving and talking to breathing and thinking. Each one of these enzymes has a unique function for which it is created. If any particular metabolic enzyme is missing or deficient in the body, it can lead to any number of serious diseases. Potentially thousands of life-supporting metabolic processes may suffer if there is a deficiency of enzymes in the body.

Digestive enzymes. Digestive enzymes assist with breaking down foods into their nutrient components for proper absorption. They are also called pancreatic enzymes, as they are primarily secreted by the pancreas, an organ found just under the lower left side of your rib cage. The pancreas regulates blood sugar levels through the production and secretion of a hormone called insulin. It also manufactures and secretes over twenty enzymes essential to digestion, including amylase, lipase, and protease enzymes, which digest carbohydrates, fats, and proteins, respectively.

Food enzymes. These enzymes, sometimes called plant enzymes, are found in raw plants such as fruits, vegetables, nuts, seeds, and herbs. By eating a diet rich in plant enzymes, you will dramatically reduce the number of digestive enzymes your body needs to manufacture, thereby freeing up energy and making more enzymes available to the body for healing. Eating plentiful amounts of foods rich in enzymes can not only give your energy a boost; it can also help reduce the energy and enzymes needed for digestion as well as boost the healing functions in the body.

The Standard American Diet (SAD) contains almost no enzymes other than perhaps those found in that piece of iceberg lettuce, slice of tomato, and sprinkling of onions found on a hamburger—certainly not enough to digest that meal and definitely none left over for healing.

Although there is little known at this time as to how we can support the production of adequate amounts of metabolic enzymes, we can improve digestion to reduce the burden on digestive enzymes. Additionally, there are two primary ways we can boost the necessary enzymes in the body:

1. Eat a diet rich in enzymes.
2. Supplement with additional enzymes that specifically work on joint healing, inflammation reduction, and other relevant processes linked to arthritis.

Before we discuss how to boost enzymes in the body, let's look at the effects of inadequate enzymes in the diet. Dr. Francis Pottenger Jr., MD, published the results of a study he conducted many years ago. He wanted to explore the damage of eating a diet devoid of enzymes to determine the effects of doing so on our body's own enzyme stores. He studied six hundred cats, feeding them a diet of food completely devoid of enzymes. The first generation of cats started suffering from "heart problems; nearsightedness; farsightedness; under activity of the thyroid or inflammation of the thyroid gland; infection of the kidney, of the liver, of the testes, of the ovaries; arthritis, inflammation of the joints; inflammation of the nervous system with paralysis and meningitis."[1]

The next generation of cats had symptoms worse than their parents. Dr. Pottenger found they were "much more irritable, dangerous to handle, sex interest is slack or perverted, role reversal, allergies, and skin lesions." Although about 25 percent of the cats born to the first generation died, Dr. Pottenger noted that 70 percent of the cats born to the second generation died. The deliveries were more difficult, and more of the pregnant cats diet in labor.

The third generation of kittens suffered from similar health conditions. None lived past six months, and as a result, they were unable to produce offspring. There was no fourth generation of cats.

For comparison's sake, Dr. Pottenger fed another group of cats an enzyme-rich diet of raw meat, raw milk, and cod liver oil, because cats are carnivorous animals. He observed healthy cats from one generation to the next. Dr. Pottenger's study demonstrates that a shortage of enzymes in the cats' diets played a significant role in their health—or lack of it.

BOOSTING ENZYMES

In addition to eating a healthy diet like the one outlined in chapter 2, the best ways to boost the availability of enzymes for healing is to reduce the number required for digestion, incorporate enzyme-rich foods into your diet, and add supplementary enzymes either to meals or on an empty stomach, depending on the purpose of taking them. I'll discuss enzyme supplementation momentarily.

Reducing the Digestive Burden

Digestion requires plentiful amounts of the body's enzymes, particularly when we eat a diet high in animal protein, harmful fats, sugars, and other difficult-to-digest foods. We eat complex meals of meat, potatoes, gravy, and vegetables (maybe!) and then top it all off with a wheat-, dairy-, and sugar-rich dessert, giving little consideration to the burden this type of meal or something similar puts on our digestive enzymes. This type of eating pattern in the Standard American Diet (SAD) is enzyme intensive; in other words, it takes a vast number of enzymes produced by the body to digest it adequately. And our enzyme systems can easily become overwhelmed when we eat these heavy, complex meals on a regular basis: think indigestion, bloating, and heaviness, and you'll have a good idea how much your digestive system may be struggling with these food choices. Check out Eight Easy Ways to Improve Your Digestion for more tips.

EIGHT EASY WAYS TO IMPROVE YOUR DIGESTION

1. Chew, chew, chew your food. Then chew it some more. As you may recall, chewing food well releases enzymes in foods. Plus, chewing well allows food to mingle longer with your salivary juices, helping to break them down further and ensuring more digestion occurs in the upper chamber of the stomach.

2. Don't drink with meals, or if you have supplements to take with meals, drink a small amount of water. Not only does drinking with

---

meals dilute the enzymes in your food and your body's digestive juices, it prematurely raises the pH of your stomach, the signal that tells your stomach to dump stomach contents into the duodenum. That means undigested foods will prematurely find their way to your intestines, where they may cause inflammation or leak through the intestinal walls—a precursor to many illnesses.

3. Simplify your meals. Heavy, complex meals like a steak, baked potato, gravy, cake, and ice cream are harder to digest than simpler, lighter ones. Digestion requires a tremendous amount of energy and enzymes; take the burden off your body by simplifying your diet.

4. Try not to eat when you are stressed out. If you are always stressed, learn some stress-management techniques—you're the only person who can manage the stress in your life. Emotional distress diverts a substantial amount of energy needed for digestion.

5. Eat prior to 7:00 or 7:30 p.m. That gives your body time to digest foods thoroughly before going to bed. If you work night shifts, avoid eating for at least three hours before bed—no late-night snacks.

6. Add a full-spectrum digestive enzyme to your meals. I'll discuss more about supplementing with enzymes later in this chapter.

7. Eat more fermented foods like sauerkraut, yogurt (preferably dairy-free options), kimchi, kombucha (a fermented tea beverage), and others. Be sure they contain live cultures. You'll find these foods in the refrigerator section of your health food or grocery store. For more information about fermented foods, check out my book *The Probiotic Promise* as well as my blog on CulturedCook.com.

8. Replenish enzymes in your diet. That means eating more foods in their natural, uncooked state.

Replenishing Our Enzyme-Depleted Diet

As you learned in chapter 2, our modern diet is replete with many weaknesses: it is high in trans fats, saturated fats, sugar, chemical food additives, sodium, and less-than-desirable ingredients. It also contains insufficient amounts of vitamins, minerals, essential fatty acids, phytonutrients, and enzymes.

Fruits, vegetables, nuts, and seeds are replete with their own enzymes to digest them if eaten in a raw, natural state. But most enzymes are destroyed at 118 degrees Fahrenheit—which is not very hot at all—and this means that the food will no longer contain all of the enzymes needed to digest it but will instead deplete your body's own digestive enzymes. Most of our foods are cooked well beyond that temperature, destroying all of the enzymes they once contained.

It's not necessary to eat all of your foods in a raw state, but you can see the problem when you eat almost no raw fruits, vegetables, nuts, or seeds: your body has to pick up the slack, depleting your digestive enzymes in the process. Not only does this result in reduced digestive function and more symptoms of indigestion; many digestive enzymes also double as metabolic enzymes that can reduce inflammation and help heal the joints when they are not needed to digest food.

Most of us fry, sauté, bake, broil, barbecue, microwave, or steam our foods, ensuring that any enzymes that may be present in the food are destroyed in the cooking process. Simply making an effort to obtain more raw foods in your diet can make a difference in improving your health. You may be having visions of rabbit food just now, but it's not necessary to eat like a rabbit to enjoy more raw foods and the health benefits they offer. I absolutely love delicious gourmet foods, and I wouldn't eat like a rabbit, but I do eat a high amount of raw foods on a regular basis.

You may be thinking that you find it hard to digest raw fruits and vegetables. If find these foods difficult to digest, you are simply not chewing your food adequately. These foods contain all of the enzymes needed to be digested comfortably and completely, but the enzymes need to be broken down to be accessible. The way to break them down is to chew them well.

Here are some easy ways to enjoy more raw foods in your diet.

- Eat more fruit in its natural state. Instead of pastries or processed sweets, indulge your sweet tooth with some delicious fruit. Enjoy some pineapple, apples, pomegranates, cherries, blueberries, and other delicious fruits. Once you make it a habit you'll find you won't miss other sweets anyway.
- Snack on vegetable crudité with hummus or a dairy-free veggie dip.
- Eat at least one leafy green salad every day. There are dozens of possible ingredients you can use to keep it interesting and delicious. To help you get started, check out the text box Create a Gourmet, Health-Building Salad in Minutes on page 86.
- Enjoy fermented foods like dairy-free yogurt, sauerkraut, kimchi, kombucha (fermented tea), and others. Make sure the ones you choose say "live cultures." This means they contain beneficial bacteria and health-supporting yeasts that boost enzymes and digestion.
- Snack on raw, unsalted nuts that have been soaked in water for a few hours. Soaking them ahead of time deactivates enzyme inhibitors found in the nuts. I set out a couple of bowls of nuts in water at night before heading to bed so they'll be ready to snack on the next day.

CREATE A GOURMET, HEALTH-BUILDING SALAD IN MINUTES

If you avoid salads at any cost, thinking they consist only of iceberg lettuce and a couple of slices of starchy tomato topped with some chemical and sugar-laden bottled dressing, you will be happy to learn that with minimal effort you can create salads that inspire health *and* your taste buds.

These excellent salads can be gourmet meals in themselves. The idea is to be creative. This list is just to help you get started.

SALAD BASES

beetroot (grated)	quinoa (cooked)
Boston lettuce	radiccio
brown rice (cooked)	Romaine lettuce
endive	seaweed (such as arame, nori, or wakami)
grated cabbage	sprouts (such as alfalfa, mung bean, red clover)
leaf lettuce	
mixed greens	watercress
parsley	wild rice

MIX-INS

alfalfa sprouts	celery
apples (sliced or grated)	celery root
avocado	chickpeas
beets (grated)	cucumber slices
bell peppers (red, green, or yellow)	edible flowers (i.e. nasturtiums, violas, pansies)
blackberries	fenugreek sprouts
blueberries	grapefruit slices
broccoli (finely chopped)	Great Northern beans
broccoli sprouts	kidney beans
carrots (julienned, roasted, or grated)	lima beans
	mung bean sprouts

mushrooms (raw or cooked)	radishes
olives	raspberries
onion (minced)	red clover sprouts
onion sprouts	scallions
orange slices	strawberries
pea shoots	sweet potato (grated or roasted)
peas (fresh)	
pinto beans	tomatoes
pomegranate seeds	zucchini (grated or roasted)

TOPPINGS

almond slices	hazelnuts (chopped)
carrots (grated)	herbs (such as thyme, oregano, minced garlic)
fresh basil (chopped)	
fresh cilantro (chopped)	pine nuts
	pumpkin seeds
fresh mint (chopped)	sesame seeds
fresh parsley (chopped)	sunflower seeds

DRESSINGS

balsamic vinegar	olive oil
oil and lemon juice	your favorite homemade dressing

Supplementing with Enzymes

There's good reason to consider adding enzyme supplements to your arthritis-proof program: they work. You can supplement your diet with a high-quality full-spectrum digestive enzyme formula that includes amylase, lipase, and protease, among other enzymes, that break down starches and sugars, fats, and protein, respectively, the major building blocks of foods. Taking enzymes with meals is beneficial for your digestion and over- all energy levels, but there is a better way of taking enzymes to alleviate arthritis symptoms and aid healing: systemic enzyme therapy.

Systemic enzyme therapy, the use of enzyme supplements on an empty stomach, is the natural medicine of the future when it comes to arthritis. The same enzymes that would normally act on the foods you eat instead go to work on reducing swelling, clean- ing up joints, eliminating the byproducts of inflammation, and boost healing of the joints and tissues. For example, an enzyme known as chymotrypsin, which normally breaks down protein foods, instead reduces swelling, is a natural anti-inflammatory, and is proven effective in the treatment of arthritis.

Drs. Wolfgang Bringmann and Rudolf Kunze, of Berlin, Ger- many, conducted a study of athletes at an official mini-marathon. For two days prior to the event Dr. Bringmann gave the ath- letes ten enzyme tablets three times daily. On the morning of the event the athletes took ten additional enzyme supplements. The athletes maintained their strict training schedules through- out the test. Dr. Kunze took blood samples from the athletes and observed that the levels of lymphocytes, a substance cre- ated by the body as part of an immune system response typi- cally indicating physical stress, were remarkably reduced, which indicated that the athletes' bodies were less stressed by their physical activity.

Dr. Anthony Cichoke cites exciting information about the effects of enzymes on rheumatoid arthritis in his book *Enzymes and Enzyme Therapy*. He indicates that rheumatoid arthritis improves or is at least delayed when high doses of enzymes are used over an extended period of time.[2] And I have found similar results in my own practice.

Jo, an information technology professional in her forties, came to see me to address the osteoarthritis she had been diagnosed with a few years earlier. She had suffered a tennis injury in her right elbow and now suffered from osteoarthritis in that joint.

She already ate a healthy diet, but we explored a variety of ways to improve upon it. Soon she was eating an anti-arthritis diet like the low-sugar, low-meat, no-dairy, gluten-free, and high plant-based diet I outlined in chapter 2. Additionally, because she rarely ate raw foods, I asked her to increase the amount of raw foods she ate, and she agreed to eat a large green salad once a day along with vegetable juices, crudités, and raw nuts as snacks.

I prescribed a digestive enzyme supplement for her to take with meals to boost her digestive functions because she indicated that she frequently suffered from indigestion and bloating. I also asked her to alternate with five bromelain and five serratiopeptidase enzyme supplements on an empty stomach every few hours, with up to fifteen total daily.

I also prescribed a probiotic supplement that she took first thing in the morning on an empty stomach about thirty minutes before eating breakfast. She found it easy to fit it into her morning routine by taking it with a large glass of water upon rising in the morning. Then she showered and got ready and then ate breakfast.

Jo returned in a month and was amazed at how much less pain she felt in her elbow. She found the program easy to stick with, and like many of my clients, the symptom improvement gave her a strong incentive to do so. As her pain levels reduced, we reduced her bromelain and serratiopeptidase enzyme supplements to three each per day on an empty stomach.

Enzyme supplements work in different ways, but they can clean up the joints, reduce inflammation, or speed up the inflammatory process so that the processes are completed sooner, which promotes healing. There are many different enzymes that can help with arthritis. Let's explore some of the main ones. Some formulations include multiple types. It's not necessary to take all of them; choose the ones that sound like a good fit for your symptoms and are available at your local health food store at your price point.

Amylase is the enzyme that helps us digest carbohydrates. When you take it on an empty stomach it has antihistamine effects and alleviates inflammation linked to skin conditions, particularly when combined with lipase. Amylase is well suited for arthritics because it increases joint mobility and relieves muscle pain and inflammation.

Bromelain is extracted from pineapple and is helpful in treating swelling and inflammation linked to injuries, surgery, swellings, and broken blood vessels; menstrual hemorrhaging; and blood clots. Taking 1500mg a day of bromelain in divided doses between meals helps to reduce inflammation.

Catalase helps relieve inflammation linked to injuries, particularly when fluid retention and edema are involved. This enzyme also functions as an antioxidant, which scavenges free radicals and prevents them from causing additional health concerns.

Chymotrypsin is effective in treating inflammation, abscesses, wounds, and blood clots before and after tooth extractions and other dental work as well as after surgeries.

Lipase is particularly good for alleviating swelling and muscle spasms.

Papain is extracted from papaya and is helpful against insect stings and can help treat inflammation linked to gluten intolerance, swelling, and wounds.

Protease is excellent for inflammation that tends to benefit from ice packs. It also alleviates soft-tissue trauma linked to accidents or surgery. Like lipase, protease is also good for muscle spasms.

Serratiopeptidase is an excellent anti-inflammatory enzyme that helps reduce swelling. In addition to its ability to help reduce arthritis symptoms and heal the joints, it is also good for reducing lung and sinus congestion.

Superoxide dismutase, or SOD as it is sometimes known, disarms free radicals produced in the energy centers of the cells, thereby improving energy production and lessening oxidative damage in the body.

Trypsin is helpful for reducing inflammation as well as treating wounds, abscesses, blood clots, and injuries.

As I mentioned, there are two ways of taking enzyme supplements: with food or on an empty stomach. Although the difference may seem inconsequential, it actually determines the effectiveness of taking the supplements to heal arthritis. Any enzymes taken with food will help digest the food; although that helps boost the nutrients that may be absorbed, which can help with arthritis, the enzymes largely work on the food with which they are taken. Enzymes taken on an empty stomach go to work on cleaning up inflammation, healing the joints, and other healing functions that help reduce both the symptoms of arthritis and boost overall healing as well.

Needless to say, it is far superior to take enzymes for the purpose of treating arthritis on an empty stomach, a treatment known as systemic enzyme therapy. However, this approach should not be used if you have an ulcer or hemophilia or for a week or two before or after a surgery. Additionally, enzyme therapy has not been studied on pregnant or nursing women, so if you are pregnant or breastfeeding, it is best avoided.

Treating Pain and Inflammation with Enzymes

Other than amylase and lipase, all of these enzymes are categorized as proteases, which means they digest protein. You may notice protease is also on the list. Protease is both a type of enzyme and a category under which all protein-digestive enzymes are classified. It's a bit confusing, but don't worry: you don't need to remember this information to benefit from it.

So how exactly can enzymes that digest protein help you with arthritis? Many of the by-products of inflammation contain a protein membrane. When you take enzymes on an empty stomach these various proteases go to work breaking down inflammation. If you're old enough to remember the video game Pac-Man, then you easily picture how these enzymes literally digest inflammation's by-products, thereby reducing pain and inflammation in the process.

WOBENZYM PS AND WOBENZYM N

One particular brand of enzymes, Wobenzym, has been heavily studied in the treatment of arthritis. It is available in two main products, Wobenzym PS and Wobenzym N. The former is the professional strength primarily sold through health practitioners. Wobenzym N is readily available from most health food stores and online.

Wobenzym PS contains bromelain, rutin, and trypsin. Wobenzym N contains the enzymes papain, bromelain, trypsin, chymotrypsin, and pancreatin (a type of protease). Both products have been the subject of a large volume of research for treating pain disorders, and both have been found highly effective in increasing joint flexibility and mobility, improving joint and tendon health, and easing aches and pains. In one study 62 percent of patients taking the enzyme formulation Wobenzym N showed improvement in their arthritic symptoms.[3]

Another German study found that the same enzyme formula prevented further arthritic flare-ups and lowered inflammatory compounds called circulating immune complexes linked to rheumatoid arthritis.[4] Bromelain, an enzyme extracted from pineapples, is also used in systemic enzyme therapy for arthritis due to its anti-inflammatory and antipain properties. There are no known drug interactions.

SERRAPEPTIDASE

Exciting research shows that a natural enzyme supplement offers help for arthritis as well as allergies, asthma, MS, and other inflammatory conditions. Also known as serrapeptidase or serrapeptase, it is an enzyme many health practitioners use as a natural treatment for a wide variety of health conditions, especially inflammatory conditions.

Serrapeptidase has shown promise in treating inflammation in animal studies. In a study published in the *Indian Journal of Pharmaceutical Sciences*, Drs. Viswanatha and Patil at the department of pharmacology and pharmacotherapeutics, Jawaharlal Hehru Medical College in India, found that serrapeptase was more effective than aspirin for reducing inflammation in animals.[5]

HOW TO TAKE ENZYME SUPPLEMENTS FOR ARTHRITIS

Supplement with one or more of the following enzymes between meals on an empty stomach: bromelain, chymotrypsin, papain, protease, serrapeptidase, superoxide dismutase (SOD), or trypsin or a single product that includes some or all of these enzymes, such as Wobenzym PS or Wobenzym N. Start with three capsules or tablets of your chosen enzyme(s) on an empty stomach twenty minutes before or at least one hour after meals, three times daily. You can gradually increase to five capsules or tablets over a week or two. Discontinue if you find it irritates your stomach.

Selecting Enzyme Supplements

Many manufacturers of enzyme supplements use genetically modified foods or bacteria in the process of sourcing enzymes. Because genetically modified organisms (GMOs) have been found to increase inflammation and have been linked to many serious diseases, it is important to avoid them as much as possible. So be sure that any enzyme supplements you choose have been certified to be free of GMOs. One independent organization grants the Non-GMO Verified statement to companies that prove their products are free of GMOs, so look for this statement or logo on the label of the product you select.

5

Natural Medicine
That Works

MAKING DIETARY CHANGES AND addressing key nutritional deficiencies are powerful ways to heal the underlying issues linked to arthritis as well as to improve the symptoms of the disease. But sometimes the body needs more support in the form of additional nutrients, herbs, and probiotics that can help reduce or eliminate inflammation and pain, heal the joints, and reverse any damage elsewhere in the body that may be contributing to the disease.

Fortunately there are many great herbs and nutrients that work well for arthritis, sometimes even better than drug options, and without the terrible side effects. Some of these natural medicines include glucosamine sulfate, methylsulfonylmethane (MSM), chondroitin sulfate, fish oils, essential fatty acids, devil's claw, willow bark, ginger, curcumin, and probiotics. Let's explore some of the best natural medicines for arthritis.

WHICH NUTRIENTS ARE BEST WHEN

In addition to the nutritional deficiencies we discussed earlier, there are many other nutrients that are important to maintain healthy joints and even improve joint health over time.

Glucosamine Sulfate

Glucosamine sulfate is known as an amino sugar, a type of compound that naturally occurs in the body and is used to build tissue rather than as a source of energy like other types of sugars. It is particularly involved in maintaining healthy cartilage and bones. People with arthritis or other joint disorders tend to be deficient in this compound, which naturally diminishes with age and as the body attempts to deal with arthritis. Supplementing with this nutrient can help cartilage formation while reducing pain levels. Glucosamine has been proven in many tests to alleviate the pain of joint inflammation when taken consistently for a minimum of two weeks to two months. In some studies it is more effective than non-steroidal anti-inflammatory drugs (NSAIDs). And in every study I have seen over the years, not a single drug can match its ability to halt the deterioration of joints and even to rebuild joints when taken in dosages of 1000 to 1500mg daily. It has been proven in over three hundred studies to build joint cartilage.[1]

Glucosamine sulfate is not a quick fix. You'll likely not notice improvement within hours of taking it—that's just not how it works. To use glucosamine correctly you'll need to take it in high enough doses to work and then continue taking it. It's not a painkiller, so you won't get relief in a matter of hours; it works to halt damage to the joints and even to help strengthen cartilage, which often reduces pain, but it takes weeks or sometimes months to really notice the improvement. It's not just a Band-Aid to mask symptoms but rather a solution to halt joint damage in its tracks. But over time you will likely notice an improvement in pain and mobility as well.

Because glucosamine sulfate is usually derived from shellfish, you should avoided it if you are vegan or allergic to shellfish. If you are suffering from osteoarthritis, glucosamine works best when taken with chondroitin sulfate, which I discuss below.

Methylsulfonylmethane (MSM)

Methylsulfonylmethane, or MSM as it is more frequently known, is a naturally occurring sulfur compound that is found in many foods. It is also naturally found in the body, but sometimes the amount is insufficient to overcome the inflammatory foods in our diet and our stressful lives, as well as any damage to our joints from injuries. That is the case for most people with arthritis: if we had enough MSM to counteract our diet and lifestyles, we probably wouldn't have arthritis in the first place. It is therefore a good idea to supplement with this nutrient. Not only does MSM improve the health of the joints and muscles it also helps to restore an imbalanced immune system, making it a beneficial nutrient for any type of arthritis, including both osteoarthritis and rheumatoid arthritis as well as fibromyalgia.

Although it is found in many vegetables, especially dark, leafy green ones, most North Americans eat so poorly that there is little, if any trace of this nutrient in the foods they consume. Besides that, once arthritis has settled into the body dietary amounts of MSM are rarely sufficient. Because we need a constant supply of this nutrient, it is best to take MSM in supplement form; doing so will not only help alleviate pain and inflammation but also boost joint health and healing.

Take 2000mg daily in divided doses; for example, take 1000mg with breakfast and 1000mg with dinner. MSM can boost detoxification in the body too, so it's best to start with 1000mg total per day and build up to 2000mg. daily. Because it has blood-thinning properties, avoid using MSM if you are taking pharmaceutical blood thinners, including acetaminophen. I'm not aware of any other drug interactions with MSM.

Chondroitin Sulfate

Chondroitin sulfate, or chondroitin as it is frequently called, plays a critical role in the creation of cartilage. It strengthens yet provides flexibility to the connective tissue found in the joints, acts as a cushion, and helps lubricate the joints. It is a member of a category of substances that are classified as glycosaminoglycans, but don't worry: you don't need to remember the classification to start benefiting from this important nutrient. Not only does chondroitin protect cartilage from degeneration; it also blocks enzymes that destroy cartilage while ensuring vital nutrients reach the cartilage for repair. Because of its work on multiple levels to prevent further joint damage as well as to improve joint healing, chondroitin sulfate is a good choice for most arthritics but may not be necessary for those suffering from fibromyalgia.

Chondroitin sulfate tends to work best in conjunction with glucosamine. Choose a sustainably sourced product because some are derived from powdered shark cartilage; others are derived from the cartilage from cows. I am unaware of any vegan chondroitin products. Although there don't appear to be any toxic reactions, some people may have unwanted side effects, particularly those who are prone to severe allergic reactions; if you tend to have severe allergic reactions (the life-threatening variety) then it may be a good idea to avoid chondroitin just to be safe. Please rest assured, however, that chondroitin is actually quite safe. In my twenty-five years as a nutritionist I've yet to come across anyone who had an allergic reaction to it—I only include this information for the sake of safety. Chondroitin is chemically similar to the blood thinner heparin so avoid using it while taking this drug or while using other blood thinners unless you are being monitored by a doctor. You may also wish to have your doctor monitor you while taking chondroitin because it may enable you to reduce your dose of blood-thinning drugs.

There are many excellent products, including ones that combine glucosamine sulfate and chondroitin sulfate so you won't need to take as many supplements each day. Some also include MSM, so you may find that you can get all three nutrients in a single supplement. Take 1500mg of chondroitin sulfate once daily or 500mg three times daily with meals.

Astaxanthin

You've probably heard of the nutrient known as beta carotene, which is found in many orange, red, and green fruits and vegetables like carrots, squash, and leafy greens. Beta carotene is one of a large group of nutrients known as carotenoids, which includes another nutrient known as astaxanthin (pronounced as-ta-ZAN-thin). Both beta carotene and astaxanthin are antioxidants that destroy harmful free radicals before they can cause further joint and tissue damage; in research, however, astaxanthin has been found to be 53.7 times stronger than beta carotene in its antioxidant abilities.[2]

In a study assessing the anti-inflammatory effects of natural astaxanthin supplementation, which measured a compound known as C-reactive protein—a measure of a particular protein in the blood that tends to be elevated in response to inflammation—43 percent of the study participants dropped from the "high risk" classification to the "average risk" classification during the eight-week study period. The level of risk measured the risk of disease linked to inflammation. Although the study group was relatively small, the nutritional supplement showed great promise.[3]

In a small eight-week study of twenty-one rheumatoid arthritis sufferers, fourteen participants were given astaxanthin and seven participants received a placebo. The participants were assessed at four weeks and again at the eight-week point of the study. Researchers found that pain levels dropped by 10 percent after four weeks and by 35 percent after eight weeks, suggesting that long-term use of astaxanthin supplementation may be helpful in alleviating rheumatoid arthritis pain.[4] Although more research definitely needs to be done, astaxanthin has been found to be beneficial to so many different functions in the body, including eye health, the prevention of brain diseases, and many other conditions, that it is worth considering when treating rheumatoid and possibly other forms of arthritis as well.

Be aware that some forms of astaxanthin are synthetically derived from petroleum products and are not recommended; instead, choose a high-quality astaxanthin derived from algae. A dose of 4 to 12mg daily is suitable for the treatment of rheumatoid arthritis. Start with 4mg daily in divided doses with meals for a month. If your pain levels have not reduced, increase to 8mg daily in divided doses with meals for another month. If your pain levels have reduced, continue at this dosage; if they have not, increase the dose to 12mg daily in divided doses with meals.

Essential Fatty Acids and Fish Oils

Essential fatty acids are critical to balancing inflammation and pain in the body because they're the precursors of inflammation-regulating chemical messengers known as prostaglandins. Prostaglandins are made from omega 3 and omega 6 fatty acids. Both types of essential fatty acids are required, but the ratio is what matters most, as you learned in chapter 2. The vast majority of the population is deficient in omega 3 fatty acids, which can cause inflammation to go unchecked in the body. Omega 3 fatty acids are primarily found in the oils of cold-water fish, such as salmon, mackerel, herring, sardines, and anchovies, as well as nuts and seeds like flax, hemp, and walnut.

Thanks to low-fat diet fads, many people incorrectly believe that fat is not essential to our body's health. But dietary fats are broken down into components known as fatty acids, which are the building blocks of fatty components of the body, including the brain and nerves, both of which are involved in regulating pain in the body.

By supplementing with fish oils you can help to quickly restore a healthy balance of omega 3 fatty acids in your body. Fish oils are among the best supplements for reducing inflammation thanks to two active essential fatty acids known as eicosapentanoic acid (EPA) and docosohexanoic acid (DHA), both of which have been found in many studies to be helpful for alleviating arthritis. These two types of omega 3s convert in the body into hormone-like substances that decrease inflammation. According to some estimates, fish oil acts directly on the immune system by suppressing 40 to 55 percent of the release of cytokines, compounds known to destroy the joints and tend to be a concern in arthritic conditions.

In a study published in the medical journal *Arthritis and Rheumatism*, Joel M. Kremer, MD, conducted a double-blind study of forty-nine patients with rheumatoid arthritis over the course of twenty-four weeks. Dr. Kremer found that the fish oils taken over the long term suppressed leukotriene B4, one of the main inflammatory substances linked with arthritis.

Similar to glucosamine, many people take fish oils and expect immediate pain relief, but the fatty acids found in fish oil go to work to heal the joints, thereby improving symptoms and overall healing over a longer period of time. Although it is possible to obtain immediate results, most people need to continue supplementing with fish oil supplements for a few months to obtain their full benefit. You may be tempted to skip this supplement in favor of options that work faster, but I encourage you not to—these fats are essential to joint healing and pain reduction, and without adequate levels, healing will be incomplete. Keep in mind that research shows that when people with arthritis discontinue supplementation, leukotriene production increases again after about one month.

So if you're fighting inflammation from arthritis, it's wise to eat fish daily or supplement with fish oil capsules daily. It takes more fish oil to lessen arthritis than to prevent it or to prevent further joint damage. Once your symptoms level off you may be able to reduce your dosage of fish oil supplements or obtain your fish oils from simply eating fatty fish several times a week. I prefer a supplement combination of DHA and EPA because both of these fats are needed to reduce inflammation in the body in general and in the joints in particular. And there's more great news: people who are deficient in omega 3 fatty acids absorb twice as many fatty acids once they start supplementing with them compared with people who already have sufficient amounts. In my experience most people with arthritis lack sufficient omega 3 fatty acids in their diet and will find that they readily absorb these important nutrients.

Take two capsules of 1000mg of fish oils daily, for a total of 2000mg per day. Each capsule should contain at least 180mg of EPA and 120mg of DHA for best results. They are best taken with food to increase absorption and to reduce the fishy aftertaste some people experience. If you take them with food and still have gas and a fishy aftertaste, you may be deficient in the enzyme lipase, which is needed to digest fats. If so, simply take a full-spectrum digestive enzyme formula that contains lipase along with your fish oil or DHA-EPA supplement.

Because some sources of fish have become polluted, look for a fish oil supplement or a DHA-EPA supplement that third-party laboratory results have confirmed to be uncontaminated with mercury and other pollutants. Although I am not aware of any fish oil supplements being made with genetically modified fish, as of the writing of this book GMO salmon was approved for sale in some countries; keep in mind that GMOs could become a concern in fish oil supplements in the future.

HERBS THAT HEAL ARTHRITIS

When it comes to healing arthritis food and nutrients are among the best but they aren't the only natural medicines that work. There are also many excellent herbs that help heal the joints, reduce inflammation, and reverse symptoms.

Devil's Claw (*Harpagophytum procumbens*)

This plant, which grows in Africa and Namibia in particular, garners its name from the large fruit that grows in the shape of a claw-like hand. Devil's claw has a long history of efficacy when used for arthritis, back pain, and inflammatory disorders. It can be taken as an herbal tea, in capsules or tablets, or as an ointment to rub on painful areas.

It works quickly to relieve pain and inflammation. Devil's claw is a commonly used anti-inflammatory and antipain herb among arthritics. Dozens of studies cite its effectiveness against both rheumatoid arthritis and osteoarthritis but research in the *Journal of Ethnopharmacology* also shows that the effectiveness drops when extracts of specific compounds found in devils' claw are used.[5] Although devil's claw contains many active compounds, including harpagide, harpagoside, kaempferol, chlorogenic acid, cinnamic acid, luteolin, oleanolic acid, among others, it is best to take capsules of devil's claw rather than specific compounds found in the plant on their own. Devil's claw, like most herbs, proves the adage that the whole is greater than the sum of its parts—a devil's claw supplement is superior to a harpagoside supplement. Whole plant compounds not only work synergistically to be more effective but also have fewer possible side effects than individual ingredients.

To combat arthritis you'll likely need to take higher doses than most devil's claw supplement packages recommend. A typical dose for an arthritis sufferer is 2500mg daily, in divided doses.

You can take this supplement with food or on an empty stomach. Some people find that taking any supplements on an empty stomach causes stomach upset; if you experience stomach upset when you take supplements, simply take this herb with food.

Devil's claw might increase the effects of medications used to reduce blood clotting, such as warfarin, so be sure to work with a knowledgeable doctor before taking these medications together. In some cases people may be able to reduce their dose of warfarin while taking devil's claw, but you should be monitored regardless. Other medications that may interact with devil's claw include ibuprofen, diclofenac, meloxicam, piroxicam, celecoxib, amitriptyline, glipizide, and iosartan, so check with your doctor or pharmacist if you are taking any of these drugs.[6] Avoid using devil's claw if you are pregnant or have gallstones or an ulcer.

White Willow Bark and Meadowsweet

Long before aspirin ever existed, the herbs meadowsweet and white willow bark were used to alleviate pain and inflammation. It was only in the last two hundred years that the pharmaceutical industry synthesized the active compounds salicin and salicylic acid, which are naturally found in these plants. The drug was given its name to echo its original herbal heritage; at that time the herb, meadowsweet, was called *spirea*. Later it was discovered that the bark of white willow trees also contained this valuable medicine.

For thousands of years herbalists have recommend meadowsweet or willow bark for many of the same symptoms for which doctors now suggest aspirin. One benefit of the herbs is that there are fewer side effects. Two cups of tea or one to two full droppers of the tincture are recommended to lessen pain and inflammation. It is not necessary to take both of these herbs, however; simply use the one most readily available or most affordable to you.

Meadowsweet appears to be less irritating to the stomach than willow bark. Aspirin is more irritating to the gastrointestinal tract than either herb.

Due to their salicylic acid content, both herbs have blood-thinning properties and should not be taken with other blood thinners, including acetaminophen, or by hemophiliacs. White willow bark and meadowsweet are not recommended for use during pregnancy. Follow package instructions for these herbs. Additionally, if you have an aspirin allergy, you should avoid these herbs.

Ginger

Ginger is perfect for more than just ginger snaps and pumpkin pie. Research now shows that this flavorful spice is better at alleviating pain than non-steroidal anti-inflammatory drugs (NSAIDs), particularly for arthritis sufferers. Considering that thousands of people die every year in the United States from the use of NSAIDs alone, there has never been a more welcome time for this life-changing news.

Avoiding the negative side effects of drugs isn't the only reason to take ginger. It is also extremely effective in easing muscle and joint pain, making it a great choice for anyone suffering from osteoarthritis, rheumatoid arthritis, fibromyalgia, or other forms of arthritis. In a study of 261 people suffering from osteoarthritis of the knees, published in the journal *Arthritis and Rheumatism*, those who ingested ginger extract daily had a significant improvement in joint pain over those who received the placebo.[7]

A study published in the *Journal of Alternative and Complementary Medicine* compared ginger extract to the NSAID diclofenac. Some study participants received a ginger extract while others received diclofenac. Both groups had similar reductions in pain, but the group taking the ginger extract had fewer gastrointestinal complaints than the drug group.[8]

Ginger has been proven effective for osteoarthritis, but it can also benefit rheumatoid arthritis sufferers. In a study published in the medical journal *Arthritis*, scientists discovered that not only was ginger effective for both osteoarthritis and rheumatoid arthritis, it was also found to be just as effective as the anti-inflammatory cortisone drug known as betamethasone and superior to ibuprofen. Ibuprofen did not work to reduce levels of cytokines, whereas ginger was highly effective in this capacity.[9] Cytokines are compounds that are initially involved in immune reactions in the body but quickly become detrimental to healthy cells and tissues, so reducing them is a valuable strategy in addressing arthritis symptoms and joint damage.

Whereas NSAIDs work on only one biochemical level in the body, ginger works on at least two mechanisms: it blocks the formation of pain-causing substances like prostaglandins and leukotrienes as well as breaks down inflammation and acidity in the fluid surrounding the joints.[10] Most drugs work only on the former mechanism and simply cannot compete with ginger for effectiveness against joint pain, particularly when used daily over months or years. In this time frame ginger helps heal the joints, not just reduce pain.

In several other studies ginger has been found to be more effective than ibuprofen (Advil or Motrin) without causing all the health issues like rashes, ringing in the ears, headaches, dizziness, drowsiness, abdominal pain, nausea, diarrhea, constipation, heartburn, stomach or intestinal ulcerations, impaired kidney function, and even death that has been linked to ibuprofen use. Compare this to ginger, whose side effects other than occasionally mild gastrointestinal irritation include more energy, improved digestion, and a speedier metabolism in people who are overweight. Ginger's track record of safety makes it a superior choice over the drug options.

These are probably some of the reasons why ginger has been used medicinally for thousands of years in Ayurvedic medicine in India as a natural anti-inflammatory food. Dr. Krishna C. Srivastava, a world-renowned researcher on the therapeutic effects of spices at Odense University in Denmark, has also conducted extensive research into the antipain effects of ginger. In one study Dr. Srivastava gave patients suffering from rheumatoid arthritis, osteoarthritis, or muscle pain ginger powder daily for a period lasting a minimum of three months and up to two and a half years. All of the patients suffering from muscle pain experienced relief, and over 75 percent of rheumatoid arthritis and osteoarthritis sufferers reported significant decreases in pain and swelling. None of the patients in this study had any negative side effects from ingesting ginger.[11] Dr. Srivastava also found that ginger has antioxidant effects that break down existing inflammation and acidity in the fluid within the joints.[12]

Ginger is one of the best herbs for addressing muscular or joint pain and inflammation, like that experienced by sufferers of fibromyalgia and arthritis. The amount used in Dr. Srivastava's study was 5 grams of fresh ginger or 1 teaspoon of dried ginger in divided doses throughout the day. Fresh or dried ginger can be added to stir-fries, curries, soups, noodle dishes, or vegetable dishes or made into tea. To make a ginger tea, simply chop a two- to three-inch piece of fresh ginger, add it to a quart of water, and boil on the stove for thirty to sixty minutes. Add one to three drops of stevia to each cup to sweeten it. Drink at least three cups daily to lessen arthritic or muscle pain. You can also add an inch or two of fresh gingerroot to your juicer when making your favorite juices.

Although eating ginger is quite helpful, sometimes you may need the faster, stronger relief that ginger capsules or tincture (alcohol extract) can provide. Take four capsules at once, three times daily until you begin to experience a decrease in pain, then reduce your dose to three capsules twice daily. Alternatively, you can take a dropper full of tincture—an alcohol extract—three times daily to start experiencing pain relief. If you have bouts of pain, you can return to the higher dose for a few days and then drop back down to the lower maintenance dose.

You can also apply ginger essential oil topically to the skin, diluted in a carrier oil because it stimulates circulation and is helpful for alleviating joint and muscle stiffness and pain. You'll learn more about using aromatherapy for healing arthritis in the next chapter.

Curcumin

Curcumin, the main therapeutic constituent of the spice turmeric, has a proven track record of decreasing symptoms of arthritis as well as muscle pain, making it helpful for osteoarthritis, rheumatoid arthritis, and fibromyalgia as well as other forms of arthritis.

Turmeric (*Curcuma longa*) is the yellowish spice commonly used in Indian food. Its main therapeutic ingredient, curcumim, has been shown to deplete nerve endings of substance P, a pain neurotransmitter. Research shows that curcumin suppresses pain through a similar mechanism as drugs like COX-1 and COX-2 inhibitors, but without the harmful side effects.

In a study comparing the anti-inflammatory effects of curcumin to the drugs ibuprofen and aspirin, researchers found that curcumin was more effective than either of these drugs at reducing inflammation.[13] Although the study was conducted to determine curcumin's effectiveness in treating inflammation linked to cancer, its anti-inflammatory results are still relevant to arthritics.

And there is more exciting news for arthritis sufferers: research shows that an herbal extract is more effective than acetaminophen (Tylenol) or nimesulide, a potent prescription NSAID used to alleviate pain. The study reported in the *Journal of Pain Research* found that curcumin has demonstrated potent pain-relieving effects, even greater than 1000mg of acetaminophen or 100mg of nimesulide.[14] Additionally, curcumin's analgesic effects lasted longer than the drugs. This new study shows that not only is curcumin an effective pain-relieving natural remedy; it also helps prevent and heal muscle injuries and inflammation. Unlike nimesulide and acetaminophen, which have been linked to liver damage and even to deaths, curcumin has a strong safety record and has even been found to boost liver function and protect the liver against damage. The study used a curcumin product known as Meriva at a dose of 2 grams per day, divided into one gram of curcumin twice daily. Curcumin also demonstrated a potent pain-relieving effect, even greater than 500mg of acetaminophen.[15] This study shows that not only is curcumin an effective pain-relieving natural remedy, but it also helps prevent and heal muscle injuries and inflammation, offering hope to fibromyalgia and arthritis sufferers alike.

Exciting research in the *Journal of the International Society of Sports Medicine* found that curcumin could also significantly decrease muscle injury due to overactivity. Twenty healthy, active men were given either a placebo or one gram of curcumin twice daily starting forty-eight hours prior to a forty-five-minute downhill running race and for twenty-four hours after the athletic test to determine whether curcumin could prevent delayed-onset muscle soreness (DOMS).[16] The study scientists chose the activity of downhill running because it is known to forcibly lengthen muscles while they are in the midst of contracting, causing a stress on the body that triggers inflammation and the production of damaging free radicals that cause muscle pain and inflammation.

Muscle damage following the period of activity was assessed using magnetic resonance imaging (MRI) as well as blood tests and microscopic cell and tissue analyses forty-eight hours after the athletic tests. Participants also reported their levels of pain before and after the running test. The scientists found that significantly fewer people in the curcumin group showed MRI evidence of muscle injury and that the curcumin group had fewer markers of muscle damage or inflammation from overexercising.

This study suggests that curcumin can help prevent and heal muscle injuries, potentially even before they settle in.[17] Although this research may seem irrelevant to arthritis sufferers, many people with fibromyalgia avoid physical activity out of fear they will experience the flare-ups linked to the disease, but curcumin may help prevent and treat the muscle inflammation linked with painful flare-ups.

Previously I mentioned that most standardized extracts are inferior to the whole herbs, but this is not the case when it comes to curcumin, which is an extract of the herb turmeric. Both are excellent choices for arthritis and fibromyalgia, but in my experience curcumin tends to give superior pain and inflammation relief. Choose a standardized extract of 1000 to 1500mg of curcumin per day, and take with meals in divided doses of 500mg at a time. Although it is possible to use turmeric rather than curcumin, you will have difficulty obtaining amounts of curcumin sufficient to repair muscle and join inflammation linked to fibromyalgia and arthritis. If you prefer to take it as food, however, you can take up to four tablespoons of turmeric daily mixed into water. You may want to add a dash of the natural sweetener stevia to make this beverage more palatable.

THE GUT-ARTHRITIS CONNECTION

When you think of arthritis, you probably never give your gut a second thought. But you might want to. More and more research links arthritis to gut health or, to be more accurate, a lack of gut health.

Arthritis has always been linked to inflammation in the joints, but it hasn't always been clear that addressing microbes in the gut could postpone the onset of the disease, alleviate pain, and even reduce or eliminate the underlying inflammation linked to the condition.

It is important to tackle inflammation, which often starts in the gut and spreads to other parts of the body. Compounds known as inflammatory cytokines, or just cytokines, are released into the blood or tissues as part of the body's attempt to heal disease. Cytokines are cell-signaling, hormone-like molecules that encourage cellular communication in immune responses as well as stimulate the movement of cells toward sites of inflammation, infection, and trauma. Although their production may initially help the body, they can quickly become destructive to healthy cells. Cytokines may affect the cell from which it originated, nearby cells, or produce effects throughout the whole body, such as with fevers,[18] or even with the body-wide inflammation involved in rheumatoid arthritis. When inflammation becomes chronic, inflammatory cytokines can wear down cartilage and bodily tissues, leading to further inflammation in the body as well as joint damage.

In an effort to better understand the effects of cytokines, researchers conducted a study on healthy adults in which they induced the release of cytokines. They discovered that cytokines, when induced in healthy adults, cause anxiety, symptoms of depression, and cognitive disturbances. They also lower an important compound known as brain-derived neurotrophic factor (BDNF), a protector of our nerve cells.[19] Getting cytokines under control is a key factor in restoring health and preventing or managing any inflammatory conditions, and arthritis is no different. Because the majority of inflammatory conditions start in the gut,[20] probiotics—beneficial microbes like bacteria and yeasts—can play a key role in addressing the inflammation that underlies many health concerns. Before we discuss the use of probiotics to address the inflammation and several inflammation-linked conditions, let's first explore how inflammation begins in the gut.

The gut has a semipermeable lining so nutrients that have been extracted from the food you eat can cross this lining directly into the blood, where they then travel to the locations in the body where they are needed for health and healing. Unfortunately, the gut can become excessively permeable, thereby allowing whole food particles, disease-causing bacteria, waste matter, or other inflammatory compounds to cross directly into the blood stream, where they can wreak havoc.

Many factors affect the degree to which the lining is permeable, but this permeability also fluctuates in response to various chemical reactions in our body. For example, when you have an argument your adrenal glands pump out the stress hormone cortisol, or when you stay up late to work or party, your thyroid levels fluctuate. These hormones cause the intestinal lining to become more permeable fairly quickly.[21]

Additionally, any time beneficial bacteria are reduced or harmful bacteria or yeasts are increased in the gut as a result of antibiotic or other medication use, stress, a high-sugar or high-protein diet, and many other factors, it can set the stage for the immune system to "sound the alarm" and increase the production of immune compounds like cytokines, resulting in increased inflammation and intestinal permeability, or "leaky gut syndrome." (Check out the text box Candida: A Hidden Epidemic for more information about a common infection linked to arthritis and fibromyalgia symptoms.) The more permeable or "leaky" the gut is, the more incompletely digested food, toxins, harmful bacteria, viruses, and fungi have access to the bloodstream where they may cause systemic damage.

If the intestinal lining becomes repeatedly damaged due to ongoing or recurring leaky gut syndrome, the damaged microvilli lose their ability to function properly. They become ineffective at processing and using nutrients we eat that are essential to digestion and our overall health. As a result, digestion becomes further impaired, and we lose the ability to absorb other nutrients our body needs for tissue and organ repair and maintenance. You may become more susceptible to immune system attacks on the substances that permeate into the blood, such as the undigested food, toxins, and so on. Your body initiates attacks on these "foreign invaders" by responding with inflammation, allergic reactions, and other symptoms we link to other diseases.[22]

It may not sound that serious, but over time this inflammatory response can lead to serious diseases as your immune system becomes overburdened and the inflammatory triggers continue almost nonstop, damaging your nerves, connective tissues, muscles, joints, and other organs.

CANDIDA: A HIDDEN EPIDEMIC

There are many kinds of harmful, opportunistic infections that can inhabit our intestines. One of the most common is known as *Candida albicans*, which is a type of fungus but is commonly referred to as a yeast infection. Arthritis and muscle pain such as that found in fibromyalgia are just two of the symptoms of a candida infection. Jacob Teitelbaum, MD and author of *From Fatigued to Fantastic*, found that yeast overgrowth is linked to an average weight gain of 32.5 pounds per person.[23] And according to some estimates at least 15 million women suffer from candidiasis–the condition caused by an overgrowth of candida. But candida really doesn't discriminate based on gender; men are vulnerable to its effects as well. The following list notes some of the most common symptoms of candidiasis:[24]

General: chronic fatigue, sweet cravings, weight gain, skin conditions (acne, eczema, psoriasis)

Gastrointestinal system: thrush, bloating, gas, intestinal cramps, rectal itching, alternating diarrhea and constipation

Genitourinary system: vaginal yeast infections, frequent bladder infections

Hormonal system: menstrual irregularities, PMS, menopausal symptoms, fibroids, endometriosis

Nervous system: depression, irritability, trouble concentrating, brain fog

Immune system: allergies, chemical sensitivities, lowered resistance to infections, arthritis, muscle pain

There are at least 150 species of fungi that are collectively known as candida, but *Candida albicans* is one of the most common ones to overgrow in the intestines. Candida fungi release over eighty known toxins that weaken the body's defenses and cause the membranes of the gut to become increasingly permeable, which, as you learned earlier, allows undigested protein molecules to pass across intestinal walls and absorb into the bloodstream. A host of different health conditions including fibromyalgia, rheumatoid arthritis, allergies, food and chemical sensitivities, and many other diseases can result.

What causes the overgrowth of candida or other microbes in the intestines? There are many factors, including:[25]

Alcohol intake (wine, beer, liquor): Many harmful microbes feed on the alcohol and sugars found in these beverages, leading to an overgrowth of harmful microbes. Beer is especially an issue because of its maltose content; maltose is a sugar that feeds yeasts and some bacteria.

Antacid use: Using commercial antacids can actually deplete your body's hydrochloric acid production, which works as the body's first line of defense against many harmful microbes, giving them an opportunity to take hold in the body.

Antibiotic use: Antibiotics destroy many harmful bacteria and beneficial ones alike, giving the harmful ones, especially those that have developed antibiotic resistance, an opportunity to overgrow.

Birth control pills: Birth control pills are composed of a synthetic form of the hormone estrogen, which has been shown to promote the growth of fungi and impact intestinal bacteria.[26]

Blood sugar imbalances: When blood sugar rises, it feeds harmful microbes. When blood sugar falls, we tend to crave sweets and refined carbohydrates, which also feed harmful microbes, thereby causing beneficial bacteria in the gut to decline and the harmful ones to take hold.

Chlorinated water consumption: Chlorine kills not only bacteria in our municipal water systems but also beneficial gut flora. Most tap water contains chlorine.

Consumption of foods that contain antibiotics and synthetic hormones: Most chicken, dairy products, and meat are given feed with high levels of antibiotics. Additionally, many animals are artificially plumped-up with hormones so the people who raise them can command higher prices based on weight. Both antibiotics and synthetic hormones throw off the body's delicate microbial and hormonal balance.

Diabetes: Diabetes is linked to high blood sugar levels, which can allow pathogenic organisms to grow unchecked and make it more difficult to contain infections.

Excessive sugar intake: Harmful, infectious microbes feed on sugar, giving them an opportunity to propagate at the expense of your health.

Hypothyroid function: A low thyroid function can be a factor in compromising digestion and the immune system, and this can cause a reduction in probiotics and an increase in harmful bacteria and fungi.

Immunosuppressive drugs (steroids, cortisone, etc.): These drugs not only interfere with your body's immune system that would normally fight off pathogenic microbes but also cause imbalanced blood sugar levels, which give these harmful microbes an opportunity to proliferate.

Insufficient hydrochloric acid production: Hydrochloric acid is naturally produced by the stomach and acts as one of the first lines of defense against harmful microbes like those that cause food poisoning. Insufficient hydrochloric acid also causes incomplete digestion, resulting in the fermentation of carbs, which feeds many pathogenic bacteria and fungi. Medications that lower stomach acid can also contribute to the problem.

Mercury amalgam dental fillings: The silver fillings in your mouth are made up of at least 50 percent mercury, which is largely released as vapors into your body. Mercury kills beneficial bacteria, thereby allowing harmful microbes to take hold.

Multiple sexual partners or sex with an infected person: Some infectious diseases, including yeast infections, can be spread through sexual contact.

Nutritional deficiencies: Dietary deficiencies of vitamins, minerals, amino acids, and essential fatty acids are needed to combat harmful microbial overgrowth. Without them, the body's immunity may be compromised.

Poor diet: A diet high in sugars, refined carbohydrates (e.g., pastries, cookies, cakes, doughnuts, white bread, and pasta) feed harmful microbes, giving them an opportunity to take hold.

Recreational drug use: Many drugs damage the digestive tract and kill beneficial probiotic bacteria.

Stress, particularly ongoing, chronic stress: Stress causes the adrenal glands–two triangular-shaped glands that sit atop the kidneys–to release the hormone cortisol, which over time can depress the immune system and cause a rise in blood sugar, the latter of which feeds harmful microbes.

Toxic exposures: In addition to mercury, other toxic metals can kill beneficial bacteria, allowing harmful microbes to take hold. Many toxins from plastics, known as xenoestrogens, also act like potent estrogens in the body and can promote the growth of harmful bacteria and fungi in the intestines.

Weakened immunity: A compromised immune system can allow harmful microbes to grow in the body without the normal immune response. Conversely, an imbalanced ratio of harmful to beneficial bacteria in the intestines can also weaken immunity.[27]

Restoring healthy gut balance with probiotic-rich foods like nondairy yogurt, sauerkraut, kimchi, and cultured vegetables along with high-quality supplements can help destroy candida and reduce any negative symptoms associated with it. Make sure the fermented foods you choose contain live cultures. This precludes any products sold in the center aisles of grocery stores because these products are pasteurized, which involves high levels of heat to destroy any bacteria present in these foods, including beneficial bacteria, or probiotics. You'll find fermented foods with live cultures in the refrigerated section of your grocery or health food stores. To learn more about making your own fermented foods or how to choose the best ones, follow my blog CulturedCook.com or check out my book *The Probiotic Promise: Simple Steps to Heal Your Body from the Inside Out.*

Candida can really only take hold if we have an intestinal bacterial imbalance in the first place, so restoring the balance is the first—and best—step to getting candida under control.

Research now links gut bacteria and the resulting gut inflammation to rheumatoid arthritis. Researchers at the New York University School of Medicine linked the prevalence of the harmful intestinal bacteria *Prevotella copri* to the onset of rheumatoid arthritis, which may set off an inflammatory response that begins in the gut and may initiate rheumatoid arthritis.[28] The researchers analyzed 144 stool samples from rheumatoid arthritis sufferers and healthy controls. They assessed gut bacteria between the two groups using DNA analysis and found that *P. copri* was more abundant in newly diagnosed rheumatoid arthritis patients than healthy individuals or those with an established RA condition.

Additionally, the researchers also found that high levels of *P. copri* resulted in fewer beneficial gut bacteria in people suffering from rheumatoid arthritis, suggesting a gut flora imbalance affecting people with the condition.

The NYU researchers built on the understanding established by earlier research published in the *Journal of Clinical Investigation*. In this study mice raised in germ-free conditions developed joint inflammation after the introduction of specific harmful gut bacteria. Study author Dan Littman, MD, PhD, and professor of pathology and immunology, said that "studies of rodent models have clearly shown that the intestinal microbiota contribute significantly to the causation of systemic autoimmune diseases."[29]

If *P. copri* infections are linked to the onset of rheumatoid arthritis and the gut flora imbalance, supplementation with beneficial probiotics that restore gut flora may help reduce *P. copri* infections. Regardless whether probiotics address the *P. copri* infection specifically, they have been shown to be effective at reducing inflammation by boosting gut health.

Because arthritis typically begins in the gut in the form of a leaky gut, inflammatory cytokines, microbial imbalances, and harmful gut infections, it can also be significantly improved by addressing gut health. Although there are numerous ways to do so, introducing more probiotics into your diet from fermented foods or probiotic supplements can be a good place to start because the common denominator for inflammatory conditions is the fact that probiotics are effective for the prevention and/or treatment of arthritis.

Probiotics may offer hope in improving joint function for people suffering from rheumatoid arthritis. In a study of thirty rheumatoid arthritis sufferers published in the journal *Medical Science Monitor*, scientists at the University of Western Ontario, Canada, noted joint function improvement in those who took the probiotics *Lactobacillus rhamnosus* and *Lactobacillus reuteri* compared to those given placebos.[30] The researchers could not identify specific clinical measurement differences between the probiotic group and the placebo group and, therefore, could not offer an explanation as to why the probiotics improved joint function. They concluded that the short duration of the study—three months—may not have been sufficient to identify the reason or reasons for the improved joint function. Similar to the situation with other conditions, because there are no harmful effects of supplementing with *L. rhamnosus* and *L. reuteri* and they may actually offer other health benefits of doing so, it may be beneficial to add a probiotic supplement with these strains to the treatment regime of arthritis sufferers.

As we discussed earlier, researchers have observed joint health improvements with the addition of *L. rhamnosus* and *L. reuteri*, so only time and additional research will tell if these beneficial bacteria can alter the course of this debilitating disease.

In a specific form of arthritis known as spondyloarthritis (SpA), researchers have extensively studied the connection between intestinal inflammation and the disease. They have identified subclinical gut inflammation to be strongly associated with joint inflammation in this condition. Although the research has not yet explored possible probiotic treatments for SpA, the connection remains. Therefore, addressing the gut inflammation with probiotics as part of an overall SpA treatment strategy may be beneficial.

Two other strains of probiotics have proven themselves helpful in treating arthritis: *Lactobacillus plantarum* and *Bifidobacterium infantis*.

Lactobacillus plantarum: **The Restorer of Healthy Intestines**. This beneficial bacteria is generally lacking in people who eat the Standard American Diet (SAD) but is commonly found in people eating a traditional plant-based diet. It is best known for its ability to reduce inflammation-causing compounds, making it beneficial in treating diseases linked to inflammation, including arthritis. It helps restore healthy intestinal walls and is a warrior against some infections.[31]

Bifidobacterium infantis: **The Natural Anti-Inflammatory**. Based on the name *infantis*, you can probably guess where this bacteria is primarily located: in the intestines of infants. However, the amounts of this beneficial bacteria tend to dwindle as we age. Supplementing with this probiotic may be beneficial for arthritics because it is a strong warrior against one of the harmful strains of bacteria believed to play a causal role in inflammatory bowel disease, *Bacteroides vulgatus. B. infantis* also reduces compounds that cause inflammation and are involved in many inflammation-linked illnesses ranging from arthritis to depression.[32]

Exciting new research published in the *Journal of Nutritional Science and Vitaminology* found that certain probiotic strains can restore balance to the immune system in cases of autoimmune disorders like rheumatoid arthritis.[33] The study found that a combination of five probiotic strains, *Bifidobacteria bifidum, Lactobacillus casei, L. acidophilus, L. reuteri,* and *Streptococcus thermophiles*, was more effective than other singular or three- or four-strain combinations of probiotics. I'm unaware of any other treatments, medical or otherwise, that have been proven to regulate an overactive immune system, particularly in the case of rheumatoid arthritis. Although more research needs to be done, considering the many health benefits of taking these probiotic supplements, it may be worth exploring a probiotic supplement containing at least 5 billion of these probiotic strains for the treatment of rheumatoid arthritis.

6

Pain Relief at Your Fingertips

IMAGINE BEING STRUCK BY an arrow in an ancient battle and recovering from the wound only to discover that your lifelong chest pains and breathing difficulties also disappeared. That is the legend behind the origination of acupuncture and its related needle-free therapy, acupressure. Wounded soldiers were believed to have experienced the sudden healing of afflictions that existed prior to battle alongside the recovery of the arrow wound. Although the story may have been embellished, there is good reason acupuncture and acupressure have stood the test of time for over five thousand years: it works. And when it comes to arthritis, it is a highly effective therapy that, when performed on a regular basis, can help relieve pain and improve your body's healing ability. Hundreds of studies now demonstrate acupuncture's effectiveness for healing many conditions. It particularly shines in treating pain.

Even the World Health Organization endorses acupuncture by publishing a list of dozens of illnesses that acupuncture treats effectively, including osteoarthritis, rheumatoid arthritis, fibromyalgia, bursitis (inflammation of the bursa of the joints), tendonitis (inflammation of the tendons), and other musculoskeletal and neurological disorders, to name a few. But you don't need needles to benefit from this remarkable healing therapy.

Traditional Chinese Medicine (TCM) includes many points on the body that can be massaged to support healing from common health conditions, including pain from arthritic conditions. You can easily massage these points on your own hands or on someone else's hands. These healing points are also called *acupoints*. Numerous scientific studies have shown the existence of these acupoints, which are located along invisible energy lines called "meridians" or "channels" that connect to various organs and systems in the body. When pressed or massaged, these points can induce therapeutic functions that are specific to each point, from reducing inflammation and swelling to alleviating pain and soreness.

Meridians are similar to rivers. If a tree falls in a river, it may disrupt the flow of water through the river and may even affect any tributaries that flow from that river. A blockage along the meridian is similar to a tree that falls in the water—it may disrupt the proper flow of energy throughout the body. When blockages occur, we experience many possible symptoms, ranging from fatigue to pain. If the blockages continue over time, we experience any number of possible illnesses, including arthritis. Using finger pressure at the points where the blockages occur helps them to disperse, thereby allowing the freeflow of energy along the meridians again. When energy flows smoothly we experience freedom from negative symptoms and better overall health.

Some of the benefits of using acupressure include

- It is free.
- It is easy to do.
- It can be done anywhere.
- There are no harmful side effects.

HOW ACUPRESSURE WORKS

There are many reasons why acupuncture and acupressure work. One of the ways is that the sensation of pressure travels the same route to the brain as pain. Pain does not only occur in localized areas like the knees or joints in the hands; it also travels by way of the spinal cord and nervous system, thereby sending pain messages to the brain. Like a highway system, numerous sensations travel the same pathway as pain, and the speed of the sensation determines how quickly the message gets to the brain. This gives us a clue as to how to control pain. Pain actually travels this pathway quite slowly. Dull pain travels at approximately one-half mile to two miles per second, sharp or burning pain travels at approximately five to thirty miles per second, and nonpainful touch such as acupressure or massage travels at thirty-five to seventy-five miles per second—much faster than pain!

Imagine it is similar to a sprint race in which runners are competing to grab a flag at the end. The person who grabs the flag first is the winner. Of course, the fastest runner will grab the flag and win. Similarly, if two kinds of sensations enter the spine at the same time, the fastest one will win, and that is the sensation that will register in your brain.

You may have noticed that when many people get injured they typically grab the injured area immediately. This is an instinctive reaction and one that works on the premise that pressure travels faster than pain and can often cut off the pain response from the brain, thereby providing relief.

Topical pain creams or lotions that create a heating or burning sensation have the same effect. Burning sensations travel between five to thirty miles per second, literally beating most types of pain to the brain, thereby lessening the feeling of pain. Of course, if you choose this approach, select a natural cream, gel, or lotion devoid of harmful chemicals and that contains a compound called capsaicin, which is derived from hot peppers, because its heat sensation tends to have pain-reducing effects.

HOW TO ALLEVIATE PAIN WITH ACUPRESSURE

Based on the same premise as acupuncture, acupressure uses finger pressure instead of needles to unblock the flow of energy that runs along the body's energy lines known as meridians. By using simple acupressure techniques combined with the dietary and lifestyle suggestions in this book, you can promote healing in your joints.

Although there are hundreds of acupressure points on the body, it is not essential to know all of the points to benefit from them. Some points are found in the area where you experience pain, whereas others are not. Proponents of acupressure often espouse specific approaches to pressing or rubbing the points, but you can get great results from doing what feels right for you and not getting caught up in theory. Most people find that holding the points firmly works well for them.

Please be patient. It may take some time while holding or massaging the points for the best results. And you might not experience it immediately afterward either. But with consistent use on a daily basis, the effort will be worth it. If you cannot press the points yourself, you might want to enlist the help of someone else to do it for you. If that's not possible, there are some good devices on the market that can help. Two of the most common are small, handheld low-level lasers, such as the Beurer laser, which is about $100 and quite effective. There are also many electro-stimulation devices that use low levels of electricity to stimulate the acupoints, such as the Pointer Plus, which is also around $100. They use light or electricity on the acupoints but have a similar effect to acupressure.

Avoid using massage oils or lotions when rubbing the points, as these will typically make your skin too slippery to hold the point for any length of time. Most people find that holding the point for at least a few minutes is best.

You can be fully clothed while doing acupressure, making it easy to do anywhere. Some of the points are easily accessible and allow you to rub them while in line at the grocery store, on a bus ride, or in the car (as a passenger, of course), or while watching television. If it is difficult for you to use your thumb or fingers to hold the points, you can also use your knuckle.

Avoid getting stressed out over whether you are finding the point precisely. Frequently there will be some discomfort at the site of the point, while other times there will not be any noticeable sensation.

Many of the points are located on both sides of the body. Hold the points on the side of the body where you experience pain. For example, if you have pain in your left knee, hold the points on the left side of your body. If you experience pain on body sides of your body, for best results hold the points on both sides. If you cannot hold the point on the inflamed or painful side of the body, holding the point on the opposite side will still produce healing results and a lessening of pain.

I included the names of the point and the organ meridian they are linked to for your information; however, this is not essential knowledge to effect results. Afterward I have described the location in words, but you can also look at the illustrations to find the area to massage. A general rule of thumb is that if you find a point on your body that feels sore, gently apply pressure or massage it—you may have discovered an energy blockage. Rubbing the area will help disperse any blockages you might have. Don't be overly aggressive while rubbing the area, or you may cause bruising.

Don't be surprised if some of the points I am recommending are not even close to the location of your arthritis. In Chinese medicine some of the best healing points are located somewhere totally different on the body, yet they are proven to be effective for healing and have been in use for thousands of years.

If you are pregnant, you should avoid using some points, namely LI4, and St 36. Although there are other points to avoid during pregnancy, they are not among those described below. Avoid using acupressure during the first and last trimester of pregnancy as well. Pregnant or not, if you are uncertain whether you should use acupressure or whether acupressure will negatively impact your health, please consult your doctor or a qualified acupuncturist first.

Acupressure may look difficult at first, but it is really quite simple. With practice you will find it becomes easier. Soon you will be reaching for the exact points at the first sign of pain. I urge you to take the initial time to become familiar with using acupressure because it is such a powerful healing modality.

Below you will find some of the most common places people with arthritis experience pain and inflammation. Choose the location(s) that are most relevant to your condition. In other words, if you feel pain in your ankles and knees, perform acupressure on those acupoints listed under Ankles and Knees.

I have listed the points using their traditional nomenclature in Chinese medicine, but don't be overly concerned that there are points called Kidney 3 or Stomach 41 or other seemingly unrelated names. And yes, if you have kidney or stomach concerns, you may find that using these points for your arthritis also inadvertently improves your symptoms of these seemingly unrelated conditions; in Chinese medicine they are frequently linked. You may also notice some repetition of the points. I've listed relevant points under each bodily part. Sometimes the same points that help the ankles are also helpful for the knees. If you used the points for your ankles, there is no need to repeat the same points for your knees.

The key to effectiveness when using acupressure is regularity. It is not adequate to do self-acupressure once per week—daily treatments are necessary, and two to three times daily is ideal. Try to take the ten minutes or so per day to improve your pain and healing with this powerful modality.

Ankles

Du 20 (Du channel). The Du channel is one of the two main channels to supply energy to all of the other meridians. It runs along the spine and over the head to the lips. Du 20 is arguably the most powerful point on the body and is located on the top of the head, about two-thirds of the way to the back of the head, directly in the middle if you drew an imaginary line from the chin, over the nose, between the eyes, and over the head. It is found in a slightly soft spot that is sometimes tender to touch.

L1 4 (large intestine meridian) is located at the top of the crease when you push your thumb against your forefinger

LI 11 (large intestine meridian) is located on the top side of the elbow, about halfway along the crease when bending the elbow joint.

UB 60 (urinary bladder meridian) is located on the outside of the leg, behind the ankle protrusion.

K 3 (kidney meridian) is located on the inside of the leg, behind the ankle protrusion.

K 6 (kidney meridian) is located on the inside of the leg, below the ankle protrusion.

St 41 (stomach meridian) is located on the front of the leg at the level of the ankle, directly centered.

GB 40 (gall bladder meridian) is located on the top of the foot, just below the ankle and slightly toward the outside edge of the foot.

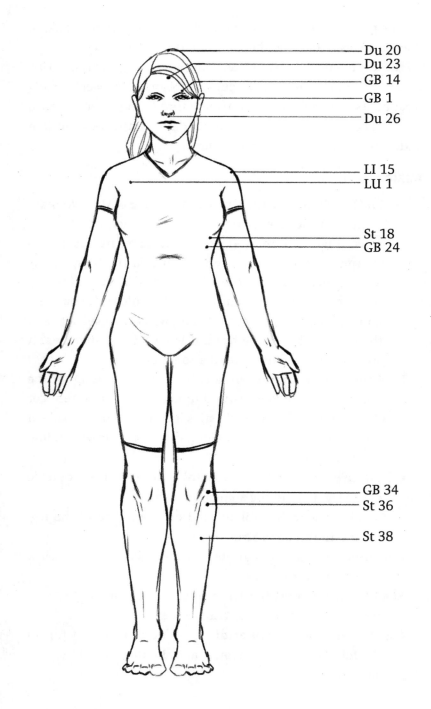

Du 20
Du 23
GB 14
GB 1
Du 26

LI 15
LU 1

St 18
GB 24

GB 34
St 36

St 38

> **Sp 9 (spleen meridian)** is located on the inside edge of the knee, at the lowest level of the knee. Use this point if swelling is involved.
>
> **UB 11 (urinary bladder meridian)** is located about one inch away from the spine (on both sides) at the level of the top of the shoulders. Use this point especially if you have degeneration of the joint or bone.

Back or Spine

With regard to back or spinal pain you can perform acupressure to help with back pain or injuries. If you have trouble reaching these points, enlist the help of a partner to rub them. Here are some of the main points to use.

> **Du 20 (Du channel).** The Du channel is one of the two main channels to supply energy to all of the other meridians. It runs along the spine and over the head to the lips. Du 20 is arguably the most powerful point on the body and is located on the top of the head, about two-thirds of the way to the back of the head, directly in the middle if you drew an imaginary line from the chin, over the nose, between the eyes, and over the head. It is found in a slightly soft spot that is sometimes tender to touch.
>
> **Du 2 (not linked to a specific organ, the Du channel supplies energy to all the meridians in the body)** is located near the base of the spine, between the buttocks.
>
> **UB 31 (urinary bladder meridian)** is located near the top of the hip region on the back, about an inch on both sides of the spine.
>
> **LI 4 (large intestine meridian)** is located at the top of the crease when you push your thumb against your forefinger. This point is excellent for relieving pain.
>
> **UB 11 (urinary bladder meridian)** is located about one inch away from the spine (on both sides) at the level of the

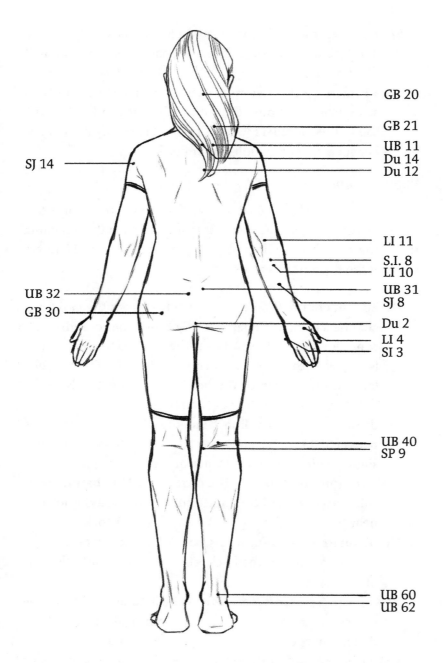

GB 20

GB 21

UB 11
Du 14
Du 12

SJ 14

LI 11

S.I. 8
LI 10

UB 32

UB 31
SJ 8

GB 30

Du 2
LI 4
SI 3

UB 40
SP 9

UB 60
UB 62

top of the shoulders. Use this point especially if you have degeneration in the spine.

UB 40 (urinary bladder meridian) is located in the center of the crease on the back of the knee.

UB 60 (urinary bladder meridian) is located on the outside of the leg, behind the ankle protrusion.

Sp 9 (spleen meridian) is located on the inside edge of the knee, at the lowest level of the knee. Use this point if swelling is involved.

Du 26 (not linked to an organ, the Du channel supplies energy to all the meridians in the body) is located on the upper lip, just below the nose.

SI 3 (small intestine meridian) is located one thumb's width up from the top outside knuckle of the hand (toward the wrist).

UB 62 (urinary bladder meridian) is located just below the ankle bone on the little toe side of the foot.

St 44 (stomach meridian) is located on the top of the foot, between the second and third toes (count the big toe as one, etc.).

Chest or Ribs

Du 20 (Du channel). The Du channel is one of the two main channels to supply energy to all of the other meridians. It runs along the spine and over the head to the lips. Du 20 is arguably the most powerful point on the body and is located on the top of the head, about two-thirds of the way to the back of the head, directly in the middle if you drew an imaginary line from the chin, over the nose, between the eyes, and over the head. It is found in a slightly soft spot that is sometimes tender to touch.

LI 4 (large intestine meridian) is located at the top of the crease when you push your thumb against your forefinger. This point is excellent for relieving pain.

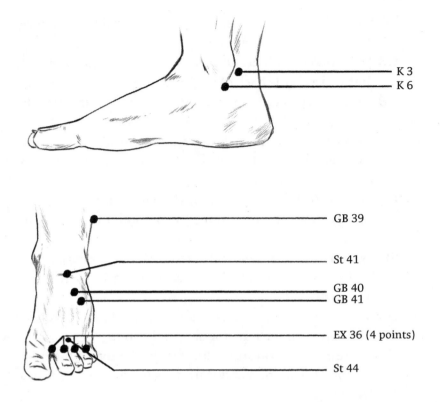

K 3
K 6

GB 39

St 41

GB 40
GB 41

EX 36 (4 points)

St 44

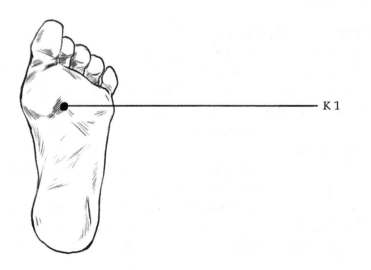

K 1

SJ 8 (sanjiao meridian) is located on the top of the forearm about one and a half hand widths up from the wrist line.

Lu 1 (lung meridian) is located on the front of the chest where it meets the shoulder joint.

St 18 (stomach meridian) is located on the chest, approximately one inch below the nipple,

GB 24 (gall bladder) is located on the bottom edge of the ribs, directly below the nipple.

GB 34 (gall bladder meridian) is located on the outside edge of the leg, near the kneecap, approximately two thumb widths below the edge of the knee.

Sp 9 (spleen meridian) is located on the inside edge of the knee, at the lowest level of the knee. Use this point if swelling is involved.

Feet

Du 20 (Du channel). The Du channel is one of the two main channels to supply energy to all of the other meridians. It runs along the spine and over the head to the lips. Du 20 is arguably the most powerful point on the body and is located on the top of the head, about two-thirds of the way to the back of the head, directly in the middle if you drew an imaginary line from the chin, over the nose, between the eyes, and over the head. It is found in a slightly soft spot that is sometimes tender to touch.

St 44 (stomach meridian) is located on the top of the foot between the second and third toes (count the big toe as one, etc.).

LI 4 (large intestine meridian) is located at the top of the crease when you push your thumb against your forefinger. This point is excellent for relieving pain.

K 3 (kidney meridian) is located on the inside of the leg, behind the ankle protrusion.

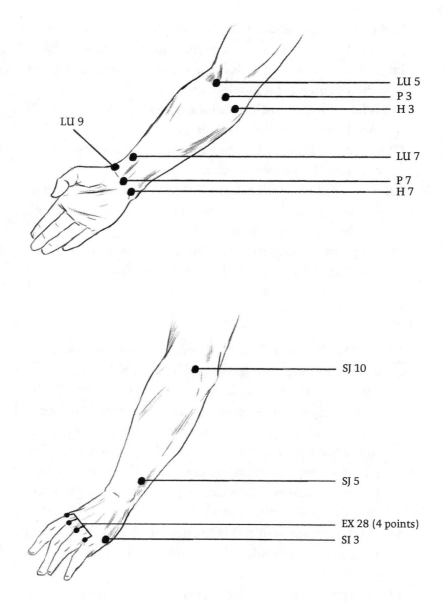

LU 5
P 3
H 3

LU 9

LU 7

P 7
H 7

SJ 10

SJ 5

EX 28 (4 points)
SI 3

K 1 (kidney meridian) is located on the base of the ball of the foot. This point is found in a slight depression.

LI 4 (large intestine meridian) is located at the top of the crease when you push your thumb against your forefinger. This point is excellent for relieving pain.

Ex 36 (extra points) are the four points located on the top of the foot where the toes join.

Sp 9 (spleen meridian) is located on the inside edge of the knee, at the lowest level of the knee. Use this point if swelling is involved.

Elbows

Du 20 (Du channel). The Du channel is one of the two main channels to supply energy to all of the other meridians. It runs along the spine and over the head to the lips. Du 20 is arguably the most powerful point on the body and is located on the top of the head, about two-thirds of the way to the back of the head, directly in the middle if you drew an imaginary line from the chin, over the nose, between the eyes, and over the head. It is found in a slightly soft spot that is sometimes tender to touch.

SI 8 (small intestine meridian) is located on the inside edge of the elbow joint.

LI 4 (large intestine meridian) is located at the top of the crease when you push your thumb against your forefinger. This point is excellent for relieving pain.

LI 10 (large intestine meridian) is located on the top side of the lower arm, about an inch below the elbow crease.

LI 11 (large intestine meridian) is located on the top side of the elbow, about halfway along the crease when bending the elbow joint.

Lu 5 (lung meridian) is located on the inside line at the elbow, slightly off center toward the thumb-side edge of the arm.

P 3 (pericardium meridian) is located on the inside line at the elbow, in the center.

H 3 (heart meridian) is located on the inside line at the elbow, slightly off center toward the little-finger-side edge of the arm.

SJ 5 (not linked to a specific organ, this meridian, also called the Triple Warmer, is responsible for balance and homeostasis in the body) is located on the top side of the forearm, about two inches above the wrist in the center.

SJ 10 (not linked to a specific organ, this meridian, also called the Triple Warmer, is responsible for balance and homeostasis in the body) is located one thumb's width directly above the tip of the elbow toward the shoulder.

Sp 9 (spleen meridian) is located on the inside edge of the knee, at the lowest level of the knee. Use this point if swelling is involved.

Fingers and Hands

Du 20 (Du channel). The Du channel is one of the two main channels to supply energy to all of the other meridians. It runs along the spine and over the head to the lips. Du 20 is arguably the most powerful point on the body and is located on the top of the head, about two-thirds of the way to the back of the head, directly in the middle if you drew an imaginary line from the chin, over the nose, between the eyes, and over the head. It is found in a slightly soft spot that is sometimes tender to touch.

LI 4 (large intestine meridian) is located at the top of the crease when you push your thumb against your forefinger. This point is excellent for relieving pain.

Ex 28 (extra points) is located in the space between the knuckles on the hand when you make a fist.

SI 3 (small intestine meridian) is located one thumb's width up from the top outside knuckle of the hand (toward the wrist).

Sp 9 (spleen meridian) is located on the inside edge of the knee, at the lowest level of the knee. Use this point if swelling is involved.

Hips

Du 20 (Du channel). The Du channel is one of the two main channels to supply energy to all of the other meridians. It runs along the spine and over the head to the lips. Du 20 is arguably the most powerful point on the body and is located on the top of the head, about two-thirds of the way to the back of the head, directly in the middle if you drew an imaginary line from the chin, over the nose, between the eyes, and over the head. It is found in a slightly soft spot that is sometimes tender to touch.

LI 4 (large intestine meridian) is located at the top of the crease when you push your thumb against your forefinger. This point is excellent for relieving pain.

GB 29 (gall bladder meridian) is located about halfway between the outside edge of the waist and the hip bone on the back of the buttocks region.

GB 30 (gall bladder meridian) is located on the side of the buttocks, slightly toward the hip bone.

GB 34 (gall bladder meridian) is located on the outside edge of the leg, near the kneecap, approximately two thumb widths below the edge of the knee.

UB 32 (urinary bladder meridian) is located approximately one inch on both sides of the spine, approximately one hand's width below the waist level.

UB 40 (urinary bladder meridian) is located in the center of the crease on the back of the knee.

Sp 9 (spleen meridian) is located on the inside edge of the knee, at the lowest level of the knee. Use this point if swelling is involved.

Knees

Du 20 (Du channel). The Du channel is one of the two main channels to supply energy to all of the other meridians. It runs along the spine and over the head to the lips. Du 20 is arguably the most powerful point on the body and is located on the top of the head, about two-thirds of the way to the back of the head, directly in the middle if you drew an imaginary line from the chin, over the nose, between the eyes, and over the head. It is found in a slightly soft spot that is sometimes tender to touch.

LI 4 (large intestine meridian) is located at the top of the crease when you push your thumb against your forefinger. This point is excellent for relieving pain.

St 36 (stomach meridian) is located in the space where the two lower leg bones meet just below and to the outer edge of the kneecap.

GB 34 (gall bladder meridian) is located on the outside edge of the leg, near the kneecap, approximately two thumb widths below the edge of the knee.

Sp 9 (spleen meridian) is located on the inside of the leg in a natural depression below the knee cap at the top of the shin bone.

UB 11 (urinary bladder meridian) is located about one inch away from the spine (on both sides) at the level of the top of the shoulders. Use this point especially if you have degeneration of the joint or bone.

UB 60 (urinary bladder meridian) is located on the outside of the leg, behind the ankle protrusion.

St 44 (stomach meridian) is located on the top of the foot, between the second and third toes (count the big toe as one, etc.).

Sp 9 (spleen meridian) is located on the inside edge of the knee, at the lowest level of the knee. Use this point if swelling is involved.

Neck

Du 20 (Du channel). The Du channel is one of the two main channels to supply energy to all of the other meridians. It runs along the spine and over the head to the lips. Du 20 is arguably the most powerful point on the body and is located on the top of the head, about two-thirds of the way to the back of the head, directly in the middle if you drew an imaginary line from the chin, over the nose, between the eyes, and over the head. It is found in a slightly soft spot that is sometimes tender to touch.

Du 14 (Du channel) is located along the spine, in the notch between the vertebrae at the level where the neck and shoulders join.

LI 4 (large intestine meridian) is located at the top of the crease when you push your thumb against your forefinger. This point is excellent for relieving pain.

SJ 5 (San Jiao meridian, not linked to a particular organ, is also called the Triple Warmer and is responsible for maintaining balance in the body) is located on the top side of the forearm about two inches above the wrist in the center.

GB 20 (gall bladder meridian) is located on the back of the neck where the skull meets the neck, about an inch on both sides of the spine.

GB 21 (gall bladder meridian) is located on the top of the shoulder, about halfway between the outer edge of the shoulder joint and the neck.

Lu 7 (lung meridian) is located on the inside of the wrist, approximately one inch above the wrist line, toward the outer thumb edge.

GB 39 (gall bladder meridian) is located on the outside edge of the lower leg, approximately two inches above the top of the ankle.

UB 11 (urinary bladder meridian) is located about one inch away from the spine (on both sides) at the level of the top of the shoulders. Use this point especially if you have degeneration of the joint or bone.

Sp 9 (spleen meridian) is located on the inside edge of the knee, at the lowest level of the knee. Use this point if swelling is involved.

Shoulders

Du 20 (Du channel). The Du channel is one of the two main channels to supply energy to all of the other meridians. It runs along the spine and over the head to the lips. Du 20 is arguably the most powerful point on the body and is located on the top of the head, about two-thirds of the way to the back of the head, directly in the middle if you drew an imaginary line from the chin, over the nose, between the eyes, and over the head. It is found in a slightly soft spot that is sometimes tender to touch.

LI 15 (large intestine meridian) is located on the upper, outer edge of the shoulder joint toward the back.

SI 9 (small intestine meridian) is located on the back, about two inches above the location where the arm meets the shoulder.

SI 14 (small intestine meridian). Place your palm on your shoulder between the neck and the shoulder joint. Reach toward your back with your middle finger; this should be approximately the location of SI 14.

St 38 (stomach meridian) is located on the outside edge of the shin bone, about halfway between the ankle and the knee. Don't let the distance of this point from the shoulder fool you: it is an effective point in Chinese medicine for shoulder injuries or pain.

SJ 14 (sanjiao meridian) is located on the back of the shoulder joint in the depression approximately two inches below the top of the body.

LI 15 (large intestine meridian) is located on the front of the shoulder joint, approximately two and a half to three inches from the top of the body.

LI 4 (large intestine meridian) is located at the top of the crease when you push your thumb against your forefinger. This point is excellent for relieving pain.

Sp 9 (spleen meridian) is located on the inside edge of the knee, at the lowest level of the knee. Use this point if swelling is involved.

Wrists

Du 20 (Du channel). The Du channel is one of the two main channels to supply energy to all of the other meridians. It runs along the spine and over the head to the lips. Du 20 is arguably the most powerful point on the body and is located on the top of the head, about two-thirds of the way to the back of the head, directly in the middle if you drew an imaginary line from the chin, over the nose, between the eyes, and over the head. It is found in a slightly soft spot that is sometimes tender to touch.

LI 4 (large intestine meridian) is located at the top of the crease when you push your thumb against your forefinger. This point is excellent for relieving pain.

LI 11 (large intestine meridian) is located on the top side of the elbow, about halfway along the crease when bending the elbow joint.

P 7 (pericardium meridian) is located on the inside of the wrist crease in the center.

H 7 (heart meridian) is located on the inside of the wrist crease toward the little-finger edge of the wrist.

Lu 9 (lung meridian) is located on the inside of the wrist crease, toward the thumb-side edge of the wrist.

St 44 (stomach meridian) is located on the top of the foot, between the second and third toes (count the big toe as one, etc.).

SJ 5 (not linked to a specific organ, this meridian, also called the Triple Warmer, is responsible for balance and homeostasis in the body) is located on the top side of the forearm, about two inches above the wrist in the center.

Sp 9 (spleen meridian) is located on the inside edge of the knee, at the lowest level of the knee. Use this point if swelling is involved.

7

Medical Aromatherapy to Ease Inflammation

DIANE, A KIND-HEARTED RETIREE in her sixties, had been diagnosed with rheumatoid arthritis when she was in her early twenties. In her younger years she could barely walk up and down the stairs of her home or complete most household chores. She had already given up her two retail jobs because she couldn't manage the tasks required due to the severe pain, primarily in her hands and knees.

Over the years she had experimented with many nutritional and herbal supplements and had transformed her diet to a largely plant-based one devoid of dairy and red meat. She rarely ever ate sweets, and when she did they were usually in the form of fresh fruit. She quit smoking many years earlier and had begun walking as much and as often as she could. Over time her joints and her walking capacity significantly increased.

Although she now led a mostly normal life with little evidence of rheumatoid arthritis, occasional flare-ups caused her to miss out on some of her favorite activities like traveling and yoga. She began using medical aromatherapy, rubbing her joints with a blend of black pepper, clove, and ginger oils every night while she watched television. Not only did Diane find the practice relaxing and enjoyable; over time she noticed she had fewer and fewer arthritis flare-ups. Plus, she informed me, the practice made her feel empowered and in control of her health and life again.

AROMATHERAPY 101

Bath and beauty companies have led most people to believe that aromatherapy is beneficial for relaxation, skin care, and bathing. Although it definitely helps in these regards, medical aromatherapy—a scientific approach to aromatherapy that uses the potent natural chemical constituents found in key essential oils—has been proven to dramatically decrease pain and inflammation, increase healing, and even restore normal pain signals to the brain—a common problem in longtime arthritis sufferers.

Aromatherapy is the therapeutic use of natural oils from flowers, plants, trees, resins, and other elements in nature that have healing properties. Aromatherapy is as old as nature itself, but humans have been using the art and science of aromatherapy therapeutically for at least six thousand years. There is plenty of archaeological evidence to suggest that aromatherapy oils were regularly used in the ancient temples of Egypt, Greece, and Rome. Our ancient ancestors must have observed that the scents of flowers, trees, and other plants had an impact on their stress levels, anxiety, sleep, mood, pain, and more.

Not only is aromatherapy one of the most powerful and fast-acting medical therapies available; it can also be a supremely enjoyable experience. Fragrant scented oils absorb through the skin into the bloodstream during massage. Alternatively, they can be diffused into the air, where they are inhaled through our nose, giving many of the molecules direct access to the brain. Thanks to our drug-, surgery-, and radiation-based system of medicine, most of us have been led to believe that medicine must be harsh to be effective and that aromatherapy seems too pleasurable to work, but because it quickly gains access to the blood and brain, impressive results are common and fast acting.

When you smell essential oils—the oil-based potent plant extracts—you're actually breathing in the molecules of essential oils wafting in the air, which send signals directly from the cells in the nose to the brain. The brain then sends messages back to the body, depending on the original message sent to the brain, which varies according to the scent (or scents) and the chemical constituents they contain. These signals then act accordingly either to reduce inflammation, relax the nervous system, boost mood enhancers, increase energy, reduce pain, or some other action based on the initial chemical constituents detected in the essential oil.

Over the last several decades research at some of the world's leading universities on the effects of essential oils on pain, inflammation, infection, depression, dementia, and many other symptoms and have found them to be effective for many of the ills we experience.

Essential oils have unique therapeutic traits and can contain over one hundred chemical constituents, each of which produces unique effects in the body. Even the same plant grown in different conditions can result in different chemical constituents and, therefore, different therapeutic effects. Additionally, each plant can produce more than one type of oil; for example, there are two types of essential oils derived from the orange tree: neroli oil from the blossoms and orange oil from the peel of the oranges. But it isn't necessary to understand the complex chemistry of the plants and their oils to reap the rewards they offer.

Oils can be divided into one of three main classifications based on their general properties: uplifting, balancing, or calming. Uplifting oils tend to boost mood and energy levels. Balancing oils tend to regulate imbalanced hormones and brain messengers known as neurotransmitters, which have a balancing effect on the body. Calming oils tend to relax the nervous system, and some even have sedative properties to improve sleep quality. I'll share some of the most effective antipain and anti-inflammatory essential oils along with how to benefit from them momentarily.

CHOOSING ESSENTIAL OILS

It is important to choose high-quality oils because the therapeutic effects are greatly diminished in lesser oils. Although there are many types of oils in the marketplace, few are produced to maintain the integrity of the plant. Avoid oils from some of the large bath and body product shops because these oils tend to be extremely low grade, are frequently diluted with other cheaper oils, and often contain synthetic ingredients. Also, avoid oils that are labeled "fragrance" oils, "perfume" oils, or "natural-like" oils, as they're usually synthetic chemicals that offer no therapeutic value whatsoever. Many of these synthetic oils are also hidden in perfumes, scented air fresheners, laundry soaps and fabric softeners, and many other consumer products, which we'll discuss in greater detail in chapter 8. Even grocery bags are frequently scented with these toxic substances and are best avoided in favor of unscented varieties.

Instead choose undiluted pure essential oils that have been wild crafted or contain organic ingredients. Keep in mind that some companies claim their products are "pure" or "natural," but these terms mean nothing, as there are no quality-control standards required to make these claims. Some companies also claim their products are "therapeutic grade," but similar to the terms *pure* and *natural*, this claim holds little if any merit.

Because essential oils are highly concentrated, a little goes a long way. It is best to use them as directed, and avoid taking the essential oils internally. Although some companies espouse this practice, doing so is best left to those with advanced medical aromatherapy knowledge, as some oils can be toxic when used internally. Also avoid contact with the delicate mucous membranes of the eyes and mouth. It's always best to dilute an essential oil and conduct a test patch on the inner wrist. Some essential oils can cause irritation to the skin when used undiluted, so only use oils that specify that using them in this manner is acceptable. For example, clove oil is highly concentrated and can be irritating to the skin when it is undiluted, but many people find that diluting a drop in a teaspoon of carrier oil like grapeseed, sweet almond, or apricot kernel oil and applying the oil to the joints is highly effective in reducing joint pain.

Some oils can cause photosensitivity, which means they can make your skin more sensitive to the sun. These oils typically include citrus and bergamot oils. Avoid using these oils within a few hours of direct sun exposure on your skin or if you know you'll be spending a significant amount of time outdoors on a sunny day. The effect typically wears off within a few hours, so you can still benefit from these oils on other days or in the evenings after you've come indoors.

AROMATHERAPY TO HEAL JOINT PAIN

Some of the best essential oils to lessen pain and improve healing of the joints include birch, chamomile, cloves, ginger, and nutmeg; birch, ginger, and nutmeg are especially good for aching joints or joint pain. Clove is a proven pain reliever (see the text box on page 151), and chamomile is excellent for joint inflammation, but there are many other essential oils that are highly effective for arthritis and fibromyalgia. We'll explore them in greater detail momentarily.

Essential oils are sold in small bottles and may seem expensive for their size, but keep in mind that you'll be using minute amounts of these oils at a time, so they'll last for long periods. Although essential oils should be undiluted when they are sold, you should dilute them in a carrier oil such as sweet almond, apricot kernel, grape seed, avocado, or hazelnut oil to apply them to your skin. Apply the oil blend directly on the injured area, such as knees, hands, and other joints or muscles (provided there is no broken skin). You can find both essential oils and carrier oils from reputable suppliers like Mountain Rose Herbals (see the Resources section for more information).

Although you can use diffusers that scent a room with the desired oils, most people find that applying them diluted in oil, cream, or ointment on aching joints or muscles is more effective in alleviating arthritis or fibromyalgia pain.

Other oils that can help relieve joint pain include peppermint, lemongrass, lemon eucalyptus, wintergreen, bay laurel, basil, ylang ylang, and spruce. Dilute three to four drops of a single oil or combination of two or three oils of your choice in a teaspoon of carrier oil like sweet almond, grapeseed, or olive, and rub on affected areas. Alternatively you can make a larger bottle of an essential oil–based liniment to use on a regular basis. Always store your oil blends in glass jars, as plastic can break down and its chemical constituents can leech into the oil. Do not use oils on broken skin unless they are specifically recommended for this purpose (most are not). Consult a qualified aromatherapist if you're uncertain about using any of the suggested remedies.

THE HOLIDAY SPICE THAT REDUCES PAIN

We often associate the sweet pungent aroma of cloves with the holiday season, but few people ever consider its therapeutic properties. Essential oil of clove, which is not the same as clove fragrance oil, can be used for a whole range of purposes, including pain relief.

Clove essential oil is best known for its ability to alleviate toothaches, making it a common ingredient in natural toothpaste and mouthwash. Additionally, it is often added to liniment and massage oils because one of its components, eugenol, has antipain properties.

Because of its potency, clove oil should be diluted more than many other essential oils: use one drop to one hundred drops, or about one teaspoon, of a carrier like grapeseed or sweet almond oil before using. Additionally, due to its potency, it can be irritating to the skin, particularly in individuals with sensitive skin. Be sure to do a test patch on the inside of your arm and wait for twenty-four or forty-eight hours to be sure you aren't sensitive or allergic to the oil.

Apply a small amount of the oil blend to aching joints and muscles on a daily basis, preferably two to three times daily, for best results.

A QUICK GUIDE TO SELECTING ESSENTIAL OILS FOR ARTHRITIS

There are many essential oils that are effective for healing joints and alleviating the pain of arthritis. The following list is not exhaustive but includes oils that are readily available and highly effective for joint pain. I've included safety information for each of the recommended oils. Remember that it is not necessary to use all of the oils; actually it is preferable that you stick with one or a blend of one to three oils at a time. I've included the Latin names of the preferred varieties of each essential oil to help ensure you obtain the correct oils and avoid using any varieties that may lack therapeutic properties or, worse, be harmful.

Birch oil (*Betula lenta* previously known as *Betula alba*) is a natural analgesic that reduces pain and inflammation. It contains naturally occurring salicylic acid (the natural form of aspirin) that is effective for rheumatoid arthritis and osteoarthritis as well as fibromyalgia and gout. Unlike synthetic aspirin, birch contains other medicinal compounds like methyl salicylate, betulene, and betulenol. Some of these substances also have antispasmodic effects, making birch a good choice to ease the pain of muscle tightness and spasms. After you've conducted a test patch to ensure you have no sensitivity to the oil, it is one of the few oils that can be used undiluted. Simply rub a drop or two into painful areas. Avoid use during pregnancy, and wash hands thoroughly after use to avoid potential eye irritation.

Black pepper oil (*Piper nigrum*): Use diluted in small amounts topically for healing joint, nerve, or muscle pain. Black pepper essential oil provides a pleasant warming effect on the joints while its analgesic compounds go to work reducing pain. It can be a bit harsh on sensitive skin, so be sure it is well diluted—no more than one or two drops per teaspoon of carrier oil—and do a patch test prior to use.

Chamomile oil (*Matricaria recutita* or *Matricaria chamomilla*): There are two main types of chamomile essential oil: German chamomile and Roman chamomile. German chamomile is the best option for its natural analgesic and anti-inflammatory effects. Avoid in the early stages of pregnancy or if you have a history of miscarriage.

Clove oil (*Eugenia carophyllata*, *Eugenia aromatic*, or *Syzygium aromaticum*) is highly effective in alleviating most types of pain, including rheumatoid arthritis, osteoarthritis, fibromyalgia, and gout. Because of its potency, use only one drop to one hundred drops, or about one teaspoon, of carrier oil after conducting a skin patch test. Avoid use if you have extremely sensitive skin.

Ginger oil (*Zingiber officinalis*): As an essential oil applied topically to the skin, ginger stimulates circulation and is helpful for easing muscular pains and stiffness and for reducing the symptoms of fibromyalgia. Use no more than two drops in a teaspoon of carrier oil. Do not use if you have highly sensitive skin.

Lavender oil (*Lavandula angustifolia* or *Lavandula officinalis*): Both a pain reliever and nervous system relaxant, lavender is good for easing sprains, muscle aches, and stiffness. If pain is keeping you awake at night, lavender essential oil is also beneficial for sleep. Avoid use during pregnancy, particularly if you have a history of miscarriage.

Lemongrass oil (*Cymbopogon citratus* or *Cymbopogon flexuosus*): Lemongrass oil is useful for alleviating muscle aches and pains like those in fibromyalgia. It also helps tone the connective tissues and can be helpful when the tendons no longer hold the joints with precision. Be sure to conduct a skin test first, as this oil can irritate those with highly sensitive skin.

Marjoram oil (*Origanum majorana* or *Majorana hortensis*): Marjoram oil can be used for easing muscle aches and stiffness along with helping to heal bruises and joint sprains. It is a good choice for topical use with fibromyalgia, as it reduces pain, alleviates muscle tightness, and helps to detoxify the area of inflammation's by-products. Avoid use during pregnancy or if you suffer from epilepsy.

Nutmeg oil (*Mystirica fragrans*, *Mystirica officinalis*, *Mystirica aromatic*, or *Mystirica amboinensis*) is an excellent oil for arthritis, as it contains analgesic compounds that significantly reduce pain. Due to its potency, be sure to use no more than one drop per teaspoon of carrier oil. Do not use during pregnancy.

Peppermint oil (*Mentha piperita*): Peppermint contains analgesic compounds that reduce pain and inflammation. Like birch, it can be used "neat"—undiluted—on the skin to help reduce pain. A little goes a long way, as this oil leaves an intense cooling sensation in the skin. Use one drop, and massage into painful or inflamed joints. Wash hands immediately and avoid eye contact.

Rosemary oil (*Rosmarinus officinalis*): Rosemary oil has antipain properties, is a relaxant, and is useful for muscular and nerve pain. It calms the nervous system, which is the route by which pain signals travel to and from the brain. Relaxing the nervous system is an important process in decreasing pain both in the short and long term. Regular use of rosemary oil not only on the affected joints but also through inhalation can be helpful for arthritis sufferers. Avoid during pregnancy or if you suffer from epilepsy.

COMFREY OIL TO THE RESCUE

Anyone with back pain knows how difficult it can be to get lasting relief. A longstanding Native American herbal back pain remedy can help, according to research in the journal *Phytotherapy Research*. Native Americans made an ointment or oil from an herb we know as comfrey, or *Symphytum officinale*, to treat bruises, strains, pain, and injuries. The medical journal found that topical applications of comfrey oil or ointment can alleviate back pain of either a muscular or joint nature.[1] Although the study only assessed the value of comfrey oil on back pain, it is effective for arthritic and fibromyalgia pain in other regions of the body.

The research showed that comfrey alleviates both pain and inflammation, and this could explain its long and successful track record. The plant contains multiple chemical constituents that are likely responsible for its pain- and inflammation-alleviating activities. Rosmarinic acid was found to significantly reduce inflammation, whereas a substance known as a glycopeptide found in the herb was found to inhibit four different pros-taglandins linked with pain. Allantoin is also responsible for comfrey's pain-alleviating properties.

Herbalists have also successfully used comfrey oils and ointments for many years in treating back pain, muscle or joint aches, arthritis, bruising, and injuries. The oil is actually made from an oil infusion–the leaves are soaked in oil rather than pressed and distilled, as in the case of essential oils. Also known as "knitbone," you can probably understand why the herb has been traditionally used for bone fractures and breaks.

To obtain the anti-inflammatory and analgesic actions of comfrey, choose an ointment or oil with 10 percent of the active ingredients from comfrey leaf (or the package might state "aerial portions of the plant" or something like that). Alternatively, some products contain 5 to 20 percent of the dried herb. Do not exceed the manufacturer's recommended exter-nal usage.

I only recommend using the oil or ointment from the plant topically, not internally, because it can be toxic to the liver in large or long-term doses or to those with preexisting liver damage. There is no evidence of any safety issue when topically using oil or ointment preparations made with comfrey and lots of evidence to support its therapeutic value. Sim-ply apply the product over the inflamed or sore area a few times daily until you experience improvement in your symptoms or until the wound has resolved.

How to Make Your Own Anti-Arthritis Aromatherapy Oil

You can make your own aromatherapy oil to rub on affected joints or muscles (the latter, in the case of fibromyalgia) as needed for pain and inflammation relief.

Here's what you'll need:

- ¾ cup carrier oil (sweet almond, apricot kernel, grapeseed, liquefied coconut, or other oil of your choice)
- 30 drops your choice of the essential oils for arthritis as listed above (e.g., you might select birch, nutmeg, and

clove, or you might prefer black pepper, rosemary, and peppermint)
- 1 small to medium glass bottle or jar with a lid to store the finished oil

Pour the carrier oil into the glass jar. Add the essential oils of your choice. Tightly close the bottle or jar with a lid. Gently roll the jar of oil between your palms to disperse the essential oils. Do not shake the oil, as it will bring oxygen into the oil, which will accelerate the oil's degradation.

How to Make Your Own Aromatherapy Joint Healing Cream

It's easy to make your own aromatherapy joint healing cream that not only helps alleviate the pain of arthritis and fibromyalgia but also won't contain any of the toxic chemicals and synthetic ingredients of most store-bought antipain creams and lotions.

If you can, keep an old blender, a small to medium glass bowl, and a spatula that you use solely for making natural aromatherapy products. Although you can use your kitchen blender, the beeswax found in natural creams can leave a residue on the blender and utensils you use.

Here's what you'll need:

- ¾ cup carrier oil (I like sweet almond oil because it absorbs well and doesn't leave a greasy film, but you can use another carrier oil if you prefer. It's available in most health food stores.)
- 1 cup pure water (or you can use rose water; available in health food stores)
- 2 tablespoons shaved beeswax (most health food stores sell plain beeswax. Be sure to avoid other types of wax because they are made of petroleum by-products.)
- 30 drops of your choice of the essential oils for arthritis as listed above.

- 1 medium to large glass jar or two or three small glass jars for storing the lotion. Canning jars work well.

Pour the oil into a Pyrex measuring cup and add the shaved beeswax. Set the measuring cup in a saucepan of water that reaches about halfway up the side of the Pyrex container. Heat over the stove until the beeswax dissolves, and remove from the stove immediately. Allow it to cool for a minute or two, but not longer than that because the beeswax will begin to harden.

Pour the pure water into your blender, and begin blending it on high speed with the lid on, with a hole left in the lid for pouring the beeswax-oil mixture. Slowly pour the oil-beeswax mixture into the water. It will begin to emulsify as you continue pouring the oil. It normally begins to thicken after about three-quarters of the oil has been incorporated. Continue adding the oil until you've incorporated all of it into the water.

Add the drops of essential oils you've selected; blend them into the lotion.

Pour the lotion into the glass jars for storing the cream. Use the spatula to remove any remaining lotion from the blender.

The lotion lasts for about six months and is best kept at cool temperatures to prolong shelf life. You can store it in the fridge if you choose to keep it fresh.

That's it. It's not as hard as you might think, and your joints will thank you for giving it healing natural lotion rather than the harsh chemicals found in store-bought varieties.

8

More Natural Approaches to Arthritis-Proof Your Life and Body

EATING RIGHT AND TAKING natural medicines to support your healing can help you feel less pain, reduced inflammation, increased mobility, and higher energy levels. But there are other lifestyle factors that can thwart your best efforts, including exposure to toxic chemicals, leading a sedentary life, and experiencing chronic stress. So it is important to address these issues as part of your complete anti-arthritis program.

REDUCE YOUR TOXIC EXPOSURE

Sadly, we live in a time of unprecedented toxic chemical use. As you learned earlier, synthetic chemicals are found in many of the foods we eat, but they are also present in the air we breathe, the face and body care products we slather on our skin, our household and office furniture and appliances, decorative items, and building maintenance products. Although it is impossible to avoid all of these toxic exposures, we may be underestimating the role of such high exposures when it comes to our health.

Many of the products we use contain a group of compounds collectively known as neurotoxins, which are chemicals that are harmful to our nervous system and brain. Although that may not seem to be related to the pain of arthritis, it is. That's because pain signals travel from the arthritic joints, through the body, to the nerves in the spinal cord, and up to the brain, where these signals are processed and addressed or ignored. Neurotoxins can aggravate the nervous system and brain cells, causing these pain mechanisms to become impaired and resulting in unchecked and excessive levels of pain and inflammation in the body. So it is important to reduce your chemical exposures as much as possible.

There are some obvious ways to reduce your toxic exposure: quit smoking if you smoke, and avoid synthetic chemicals in your food and beverages. Additionally, it's important to make the switch to more natural personal care and household products. Let's explore some of the worst offenders.

The "Dirty Dozen" Toxins in Your Skincare Products and Cosmetics

There are more than eighty-two thousand chemicals in common cosmetics and personal care products.[1] Because the skin is the body's largest detox organ and one of the best ways to eliminate toxins is through perspiration, slathering chemicals on your skin may actually impair proper skin detoxification and increase the number of toxins absorbed into your body.

It's more important than ever to read labels on your skincare products and cosmetics. Avoid products that contain what I call the Dirty Dozen skincare toxins. If your products don't have labels, it's fair to assume the manufacturer has something to hide and these products are best avoided. Although not all of these chemicals have been tested for their ability to cause inflammation and pain, it's best to stay away from them all. Many of these chemicals are also known hormone disruptors, most of which cause a condition known as estrogen dominance, in which the ratio of estrogen is excessively high in comparison to other hormones in the body such as progesterone. Estrogen dominance has also been linked to joint pain.[2] Here are the toxic chemicals I that make my Dirty Dozen list:[3]

Artificial dyes and coal tar: These numbered dyes have names like yellow dye #5 or red dye #4 and are found in most cosmetics, body care products, and hair dyes. Derived from coal tar, they also sometimes appear on the label as "CI" followed by five numbers such as "CI 75000." They contain heavy metals that are toxic to the brain and are potential carcinogens.

Benzoates: Often these chemicals go by the name benzyl- or sodium benzoate. In the presence of vitamin C, which is almost always present in the body, they form benzene, a highly inflammatory and carcinogenic substance.

BHA and BHT: The full name of these chemicals are butylated hydroxyanisole and butylated hydroxytoluene. Both of these chemicals are suspected carcinogens and hormone disruptors. When hormones become imbalanced they frequently contribute to inflammation.

DEA, MEA, and TEA: The full names of these chemicals that make products sudsy or creamy are diethanolamine, monoethanolamide, and ethanolamine. These toxic ingredients react to form nitrosamines that are both inflammatory and cancer causing.

Dibutyl phthalate: Found in cosmetics and baby-care products, phthalates have been linked to asthma, birth defects, and cancer. Phthalates are linked to impaired cellular communication, which can cause any number of health problems.

Fragrance: The single ingredient "fragrance" or "parfum" can actually contain up to five hundred other ingredients, many of which are petroleum by-products and have been linked to cancer, asthma, allergies, and nerve damage. I have personally observed a flare-up of pain levels when I've been exposed to perfumes and fabric softeners containing them.[4]

Lead: Lead is rarely listed but frequently found in cosmetics, especially lipsticks, so be sure yours says "lead-free." Lead is a serious threat to the brain and nervous system and is difficult to eliminate once it gets absorbed into the body.

Parabens: Used to extend the shelf life of products, these toxins go by many names, including butyl-, ethyl-, isobutyl-, methyl-, and propyl-parabens. The European Commission on Endocrine Disruption have identified parabens as hormone disruptors and a contributing cause of hormonally linked cancer, reproductive disorders, and other serious health issues.[5]

Petrolatum: Found in many products including "petroleum jelly," it is derived from petroleum products, many of which are known hormone disruptors.

Sodium lauryl sulphate: Acts as a foaming agent and is frequently found in shampoo, body wash, and soap, and it may cause cancer.[6]

Stearalkonium chloride: A common allergen found in many conditioners and creams. Often cited as "natural," it is a toxic ingredient that is used because it is cheaper than natural protein ingredients.

Toluene: Found in nail polish, toluene is an extremely toxic ingredient that can cause damage to the nervous system, blood, eye, liver, kidney, and respiratory system. It may also affect a developing fetus.

Triclosan: Added to cosmetics and body-care products as an antibacterial ingredient, it is contributing to the development of virulent superbugs resistant to our best drugs. Because rheumatoid arthritis has been linked to infectious bacteria, it is important to avoid substances that can make these infections more difficult to address.

How to Detox Your Skin Care Products and Cosmetics

Although it is impossible to avoid all toxic ingredients, our toxic load is way too high, and we should take measures to reduce it. Start by reading labels on your cosmetics. No ingredient list? Sorry, but the company probably has something to hide. Avoid products without ingredient lists. If you see some of the ingredients I've listed above, skip the product altogether. Switch to natural products, but remember that just because you found it at your health food store doesn't mean it's healthy. The cosmetic industry has bastardized the words "organic" and "natural," and as such, those terms don't necessarily mean fewer toxic ingredients. It is imperative to read labels and choose those devoid of these substances. It gets easier with practice.

Switch Your Perfume and Air Fresheners

If you've walked through a department store lately, you may have been overwhelmed by the perfume section. Whether you are obsessed with Obsession, a believer in Believe, or consumed by L'Air du Temps, the smell of perfumes and colognes can be overwhelming. Unfortunately the toxic effects of fragrances can also be overwhelming.

As I mentioned earlier, there are over five hundred potential chemicals that can be used under the single name "fragrance" found on the label of many products, not just perfumes and colognes. Fragrances are found in air fresheners, room deodorizers, cosmetics, fabric softeners, laundry detergents, candles, and many other products. Manufacturers are not required to list ingredients on the labels of these products, nor do they need to reveal the specific ingredients that qualify as "fragrance" to regulating authorities because they are protected as trade secrets.

Some of the most common chemicals in perfumes are ethanol, acetaldehyde, benzaldehyde, benzyl acetate, a-pinene, acetone, benzyl alcohol, ethyl acetate, linalool, a-terpinene, methylene chloride, styrene oxide, dimenthyl sulphate, a-terpineol, camphor, and limonene. Some of these chemicals cause joint aches and muscle pain in people suffering from arthritis and fibromyalgia, and even those who do not have these conditions are vulnerable. Additionally, they have been found to cause irritability, mental vagueness, asthma, bloating, joint aches, sinus pain, fatigue, sore throat, eye irritation, gastrointestinal problems, laryngitis, headaches, dizziness, swollen lymph nodes, spikes in blood pressure, coughing, and burning or itching skin irritations.

Research confirms that many of the ingredients in fragrances are neurotoxins, meaning that they have poisonous effects on the brain and nervous system. Additional studies link other negative emotional, mental, and physical symptoms to various fragrance ingredients. Until recently, scientists believed an impermeable mechanism known as the "blood-brain barrier" protected the brain. But recent studies show that this system allows many environmental toxins, including those found in perfumes and other scented products, access to the delicate brain, and that once they enter the brain, the body can take decades to eliminate them—decades that can result in inflammation.

And that's just the tip of the iceberg. Acetaldehyde is a probable human carcinogen. In animal studies it crossed the placenta to an unborn fetus. The chemical industry's own Toxic Data Safety Sheets list headaches, tremors, convulsions, and even death as a possible effect of exposure to acetonitrile, another common fragrance ingredient. In other animal studies styrene oxide causes depression. Toluene (also known as methyl benzene) is a well-established neurotoxin that can cause loss of muscle control, brain damage, headaches, memory loss, and problems with speech, hearing, and vision—many symptoms that mimic brain diseases. Musk tetralin (AETT) has been shown to actually cause brain cell and spinal cord degeneration.

Some fragrance ingredients disrupt our natural brain hormonal balance, causing any number of possible emotional concerns, including anxiety, mood swings, and depression. Feeling achy or down? It could be the scent you're wearing.

Most commercial brands of perfumes and colognes contain harmful synthetic chemicals. These toxic chemicals are not only found in many perfumes and colognes; they are also found in air fresheners and deodorizers, laundry soap, fabric softeners, scented candles, and other scented products.

If you're still not convinced these commonly available products are putting your joints at risk, here are eight neurotoxins found in most fabric softeners (and eight reasons to switch to natural options.)

1. **Alpha-Terpineol** is a chemical that has been linked to disorders of the brain and nervous system.
2. **Benzyl acetate** has been linked to cancer of the pancreas.
3. **Benzyl alcohol** has been linked to headaches, nausea, vomiting, dizziness, depression, as well as disorders of the brain and nervous system.
4. **Chloroform** is on the Environmental Protection Agency's Hazardous Waste list because it has been identified as a carcinogen and neurotoxin, which means it is toxic to the brain and nervous system.
5. **Ethanol** is also on the EPA's Hazardous Waste list for its ability to cause brain and nervous system disorders.

6. **Ethyl Acetate** causes headaches and is on the EPA Hazardous Waste list
7. **Linalool** this chemical caused loss of muscle coordination, nervous system and brain disorders, and depression in studies.
8. **Pentane** causes headaches, nausea, dizziness, fatigue, drowsiness, and depression.

The standard argument in favor of using fabric softeners is that the amount of the chemicals to which a person is exposed is insufficient to cause harm. Studies, however, are showing that even minute amounts of these toxins can have serious effects. So think twice before you add that dryer sheet or liquid fabric softener to your laundry.

Shakespeare claimed, "That which we call a rose by any other name would smell as sweet." But thanks to today's chemical industry, that is no longer true. Worse than that, the potential brain health effects are anything but sweet.

Switch your perfume to an all-natural essential oil blend. Originally perfumes were made from essential oils; they were only relatively recently changed to be cheaper chemical varieties. Perfumes or colognes made exclusively from essential oils are not only a healthier option; they smell better too. So while you're selecting a natural essential oil, be sure to stop using "air fresheners," "air sanitizers," and "air deodorizers." Even many "natural" or "unscented products" simply use extra ingredients to mask the scents, so be sure to choose unscented varieties or read the labels on products you've selected at your local health food store, as they tend to be superior to many grocery store varieties.

Choose laundry soap and natural alternatives to dryer sheets at your local health food store as well. You can add a half cup of baking soda to the water in your washing machine prior to adding laundry as a natural alternative to fabric softener. Not only will your brain thank you, but your pocketbook will as well.

And like I tell my clients, once you've had a break from the chemical versions you'll never go back. Most people find their sense of smell improves and after about a month or more of being chemical scent-free, they actually find the scents they once loved revolting.

STRENGTHENING, STRETCHING, BREATHING, AND HEALING

Exercise is critical to your success in healing from arthritis or fibromyalgia—the *right* exercise, that is. Sometimes you may need to rest your joints instead of exercise, but gentle exercise to strengthen the joints and muscles can help oxygenate tissues to improve healing and rebuild the joints. Begin gradually and work up to doing more exercise. Remember, when it comes to arthritis and fibromyalgia, there is no such thing as "no pain, no gain." At the first sign of pain stop what you are doing because you may add insult to injury. Prior to starting any new exercise program, particularly those sustained after joint injuries, it is important you check with your doctor.

Exercise benefits you in many ways, including:

- increases energy
- reduces stress
- burns fat
- speeds metabolism
- builds bone mass
- increases oxygen to the tissues and organs
- builds muscle
- improves posture
- improves lung capacity and strength
- increases flexibility
- strengthens joints
- balances the spine and hips

- increases bodily awareness
- balances the brain
- calms the mind
- greater relaxation
- improves self-confidence
- facilitates weight loss or gain (as needed)

These are just some of the health benefits of exercise. Keep in mind that not all types of exercise offer all of the above benefits. Each form of exercise has its own benefits.

There are many types of exercise, many of which are helpful for healing arthritis and fibromyalgia. Some excellent forms of exercise that offer many of the above benefits and are suitable for your healing program include walking, qigong, yoga, Pilates, strength training, and breathing exercises. These types of exercises offer many of the above-mentioned benefits.

Walk Your Way to Pain-Free Joints

Consider some of the advantages of walking to help you heal your joints:

- It reduces the risk of cancer, heart disease, and stroke.
- It has a very low injury-risk level.
- It decreases the risk of diabetes by improving your body's ability to use insulin.
- It helps prevent osteoporosis by strengthening your bones.
- It can help you lose weight, sleep better, reduce stress and depression, and ease PMS and menopausal symptoms.
- It is safer than running. Half of all runners, recreational or competitive, develop injuries such as knee and hip problems, stress fractures, shin splints, and lower back problems. Walking is much easier on the body.

Walking for fitness should be faster than a stroll. If a stroll takes about eight minutes to complete a kilometer, then walking for fitness should be between five and six minutes to complete a kilometer. Begin gradually after your injury and eventually work up to that pace.

Be aware of your posture when walking. Hold your body tall and erect, with your head up and your chin pulled back. Let go of any tension in your neck and shoulders. Pull in your abdomen and buttocks to lengthen and straighten your spine.

Are you suffering from achy joints linked to osteoarthritis? You'll be happy to know you might be able to walk it off, according to researchers at Northwestern University in Chicago. In their study published in the journal *Arthritis Care and Research* they found that for every one thousand steps a person takes, he or she can reduce knee pain and physical limitation by about 18 percent; they estimate that to be about one-half mile.[7] And the pain diminishes the longer you walk—to a point, of course. The researchers explain that walking strengthens joint-protective muscles and encourages the release of pain-reducing chemicals produced by the body, helping to keep knees healthier and stronger.

It's easy to stop walking and become more sedentary as joint pain settles in. But simply being less sedentary improves physical function and reduces pain at the same time.

Unlike rheumatoid arthritis, which is an autoimmune disorder in which the body's immune system attacks its own joints, osteoarthritis is frequently the result of joint damage caused by injuries. The most obvious symptom of unhealthy joints is pain. Other symptoms can include joint stiffness, buckling or instability, diminished function (reduced range of motion) of the joint, enlargement of the bones around the joint, tenderness when the joint is touched, heat or excess fluid in the joint, and/or deformity of the joint. If you are suffering from any of these symptoms, you should get checked by your physician.

Qigong for Great Joint Health

Qigong (pronounced chee-gung) is an integrated mind-body healing method that has been practiced in China for thousands of years and is gaining popularity in the West. *Qi* is the Chinese word for "life energy," and *gong* can be translated as "work" or "benefits acquired through perseverance and practice," according to Ken Cohen, one of the foremost Western practitioners of qigong. It is a holistic system of self-healing exercises and meditation, focusing primarily on breathing techniques, movement, self-massage, and posture.

The purpose of qigong is:

• to improve energy circulation through the entire body;
• to replace impure or diseased "chi" with pure, healing "chi"; and
• to improve overall health and well-being.

I find qigong an excellent form of exercise for anyone, but even people who have suffered very serious injuries or have terrible joint pain find they can benefit from this gentle but powerful activity. Don't be fooled by how easy it appears; qigong offers countless healing benefits that make it a worthy pursuit. Even if you can't do the standing postures, you can do it sitting.

There are two main types of qigong: active or dynamic, and tranquil or passive. Active is the more commonly seen type, involving full or partial body movements in a series of postures, held or repeated for different lengths of time. Passive qigong is more like meditation, with a specific focus on controlling the qi through mental concentration and visualization while the body is still. In short, active is exercise; passive is meditation. Anyone can practice qigong, including young children and elderly people, people with no health problems or people with serious disabilities. It can be practiced standing, sitting, or lying down.

Both forms are effective for healing arthritis. You can join a class or follow along with a video.

Yoga to Stretch Your Joints

Yoga comes from the Sanskrit word *yug*, which means "to join together." It is more than just stretching; it also advocates a holistic approach to healthful living through ethical practice, physical exercises (known as *asans*), breathing exercises (known as *pranayama*), and meditation training.

Asans, or stretching exercises, are designed to develop maximum flexibility and strength in the skeletal, muscular, and nervous systems, with a special emphasis on a strong and supple spine. The exercises also serve to massage internal organs, improve circulation, and increase oxygen and its distribution throughout the body and the brain at the cellular level. Yoga stretches and relaxes the body, calms the mind and emotions, and aids recovery from all forms of accumulated stress.

Studies show that yoga reduces muscular tension and blood pressure, improves oxygen intake, circulation, digestion, and elimination; regulates metabolism and the working of all the glands and organs; and enhances the function of the nervous system for increased calmness and energy. It is therapeutic for people healing from arthritis.

There are many excellent yoga classes and videos. Choose one for beginners or, if you can, for those suffering from joint injuries or arthritis. Be careful not to overstretch your joints so you avoid injury or aggravation of your joint symptoms. Your joints should never be in a "locked" position but instead should keep a slight bend in them.

Pilates for Powerful Joint Health

Named after its founder, Joseph Pilates, Pilates is a unique combination of exercises to be performed in a specific order. In this way you are able to balance your body's structure, strengthen muscles, and lengthen your body. Pilates was designed specifically for healing from injuries, making it a perfect form of exercise for those suffering from the early stages of arthritis. Some of the exercises can be rather intense, so it may not be suitable for those with advanced arthritis. Be sure to consult a doctor before undertaking Pilates.

Joseph Pilates (born in 1880 in Germany) studied the human physiology and ways to improve it; modern research has since confirmed his insights. He developed a practice in New York helping athletes recover from injuries. The main premise of Pilates is that it relies on building up your *powerhouse*—abdominal, lower back, buttock, and inner thigh muscles. In turn, these muscles help realign your spine and the rest of your body, helping it to heal from injuries and making it less prone to further injury.

Pilates helps develop flexibility, realign your body, enhance mental alertness, increase blood supply throughout your body, decrease stress and tension, boost breathing capacity, and improve body shape and posture.

You gain maximum benefit when you practice Pilates exercises four times per week, but you will still reap many rewards if you do less. Consider joining a beginner's or gentle Pilates class or following along with a video.

Improve Joint Health Through Posture

Along with any stretching or strengthening program, it is a good idea to focus on improving your posture. Most people have poor posture and need a reminder to improve it: we may slouch when we sit, hunch when walking or standing, lean our neck forward, and tilt our feet inward or outward. Although we may not have noticed the toll poor posture takes on our health when we are well, it becomes essential to immediately pay attention and correct poor postural patterns when joint damage occurs.

Poor posture can significantly increase the pressure on the joints, making them more vulnerable to damage. Additionally, poor posture can cause tension along the length of the spine, resulting in pain in the neck, shoulders, back, hips, and legs. It can also be implicated in headaches and restrictive breathing. It can reduce the circulation of blood and oxygen that alleviates inflammation and tension, not to mention lessen the blood and oxygen to organs and glands.

Two occupational therapists in New York City, Jane Gatanis and Alyssa Frey, have developed a powerful pain-reduction program; part of this program addresses incorrect posture. The Body Alignment Exercise takes less than a minute to perform and helps align posture and deepen your breathing. With repeated use it will make you more aware of the various parts of your body and how your body feels, and you will feel more in control of the pain and tension. They recommend beginning by practicing the exercise five times per day for the first two weeks and then three times per day afterward. It can be done almost anywhere, even while waiting in line at the bank. If you are able to stand, here's how to perform this simple exercise:

1. Stand with your feet firmly planted about six inches apart. Keep your ankles parallel to each other and your slightly bent knees facing forward. Try to keep your weight evenly distributed on your feet. Gatanis and Frey suggest visualizing that your big toe, little toe, and heel are a stool that bears your weight evenly.
2. With your arms at your sides, position your hands with your palms facing forward, allowing your chest to be more open.
3. Using your lower abdominal muscles, gently pull your belly upward and inward. Your abdomen should only slightly flatten. Don't shift the position of your back unnaturally. Hold for five to ten seconds, breathing normally.
4. Drop your shoulders downward and toward the back and lift your chest slightly.

5. Visualize your head floating over your spine. Move your chin slightly back toward your neck and chest.
6. Breathe in deeply to the count of five, and exhale to the count of five. As you inhale, relax your upper abdominal muscles so the lower parts of your lungs fill with fresh air.

Deep Breathing to Boost Joint and Muscle Health

Even if physical exercise is too difficult, you can engage in deep breathing exercises to boost your health and healing. Remember that every tissue, muscle, and joint needs adequate oxygenated blood to heal. Breathing deeply is one of the best ways to boost oxygen flow throughout your blood. It costs nothing, requires no special skills or equipment, and is available to everyone. Here is a simple deep breathing exercise to get you started. The more frequently you practice it, the greater the results.

1. Take several deep breaths, focusing on your breath's natural rhythm.
2. Begin breathing into your solar plexus area—which is found in the center of the abdominal area just below where the rib cage splits apart—visualizing it becoming warm and relaxed.
3. Continue breathing in and out into the solar plexus area for at least five minutes.
4. Repeat this breathing exercise throughout the day.

Exercise does not have to be difficult or tedious to be effective. It is important to enjoy whatever exercise you do—you will reap greater benefits that way. Add music and variety to your exercise to ensure it is fun as well.

Stress hormones can worsen pain and inflammation, so it is important to practice stress management through exercises like walking, qigong, yoga, and breathing exercises. Of course, a positive attitude is also helpful. In many studies researchers have found that stress or a negative outlook can greatly diminish healing ability, depress the immune system, increase damaging hormones, and decrease energy. Although you may not always feel great about having arthritis or fibromyalgia or the way it may prevent you from doing certain activities, it is important to allow yourself to feel those feelings and then move on to allow your body to heal.

RELEASE THE STRESS

There are many effective ways to release feelings of stress, including confiding in a partner or close friend, writing the feelings out, or crying if you need to. Recognize that you are simply feeling down for a moment in time, a moment that can just as easily be turned around to create a positive outlook. Make sure you eliminate or reduce whatever stress you can.

Additionally, start a gratitude journal: every day write down ten things for which you are grateful. Do not repeat the same things from one day to the next. Try to keep this journal going for at least a month, and you'll likely notice that your attitude becomes more positive and health promoting.

Ensure you get enough sleep. If pain is affecting your sleep, try the foods and remedies I suggested earlier. Here are some of my favorite sleep-improving strategies:

- Avoid eating at least three hours before bed, as indigestion, bloating, or heartburn can interfere with your ability to fall asleep. Definitely skip the caffeine in the evening or any time after 3 p.m. if you have difficulty sleeping.
- Get into a regular evening relaxation ritual: dim the lights, stop working, take a bath, or do something relaxing before bedtime.

- Unplug electronic devices or any blue-light emitting appliances like televisions, smartphones, computers, and so forth because the blue light can interfere with sleep cycles. If you need a night light, choose a red bulb for it, as red light doesn't seem to interfere with the body's ability to fall into a deep state of sleep.
- Stop working at least a few hours before bed. Avoid other mentally stimulating activities too close to bedtime.
- Go to sleep at the same time each night. Your body will start to adjust to these patterns, helping you to feel sleepy when your bedtime approaches.
- Use lavender oil. Alan R. Hirsch, MD, author of *Life's a Smelling Success*, found that smelling pure lavender calmed the entire nervous system in only a minute, helping people to feel more relaxed and sleepier. Sniff some lavender essential oil or flowers, or spray lavender water on your pillowcase (water only, because the oil may stain). Be sure to choose organic lavender oil, not fragrance oil, because the latter has no health benefits and may contain toxic substances.
- Take a warm, therapeutic bath. Here are two types of healing baths to consider using as part of your day-to-day health regime.
  1. Every day soak in a warm bath with a half cup of baking soda added to the water. This alkalises the water that, in turn, helps alkalize your blood. Slightly alkaline blood enables the body to heal faster, reducing pain and inflammation. Soak for at least twenty minutes. If you have excessive inflammation, you may want to wait until some of the swelling dissipates before immersing the area into warm water.
  2. Before retiring to bed, dissolve about one pound of Epsom salts into a warm bath. Soak for about twenty minutes. When you are finished, do not rub yourself

dry; instead, wrap yourself in several warm towels and go to bed immediately. This will help your body detoxify and heal.

Arthritis is a complex disease that requires a broad-spectrum approach to healing. It is not what a person does periodically that matters but what a person does consistently to help his or her body heal over time. The adage that "patience is a virtue" may never have been truer than with a chronic disease like arthritis. Patience and persistence are the keys to a pain-free life and great health.

9

Recipes for Relief

EATING FOR HEALING IS easier and tastier than you might think. It includes plenty of fruits and vegetables prepared in gourmet dishes that not only help your body heal but also taste fabulous. Some of these recipes are among my favorites, so don't let their healthy nature put you off. You'll discover some real treasures among them, and I'm sure some of these recipes are sure to become your favorites as well.

Make the main dish a large, raw salad. Eat cooked food as a complement. It is actually quite simple once you make this eating pattern habitual.

In this chapter you'll find make-at-home recipes for foods and beverages that relieve pain, reduce inflammation, and heal joints. Some of the recipes include Dr. Cook's Ginger Pain-Relief Tea, Anti-Inflammatory Juice, Happy Joint Juice, Anti-Arthritis Powerhouse Salad, and Ultimate Joint-Healing Curry. Enjoy!

JUICES, SMOOTHIES, AND TEAS

Anti-Inflammatory Juice

> 6 large carrots (remove tops), chopped into large chunks
> 1 apple, chopped into large chunks
> 1-inch piece ginger

Pass all of the ingredients through a juicer. Drink immediately.

Pain-Busting Juice

> ½ pineapple, outer skin removed (juice the core as well as
>   the flesh), chopped into large chunks
> 1-inch piece ginger

Pass all of the ingredients through a juicer. Dilute with pure water to taste. Drink immediately.

Blood-Cleansing Juice

Dandelion is useful for cleansing the blood, which removes toxins from the tissues and joints, thereby speeding healing and lessening pain and inflammation. Be aware that if you drink a fair amount of this juice over a short period of time, it can speed a cleansing reaction, which initially might produce symptoms like fatigue or headaches. These will pass as your body becomes "cleaner."

> 3 apples, chopped into large chunks
> handful of fresh dandelion (if you are digging it yourself, be
>   sure to obtain organic dandelion, where the land has not
>   been sprayed for several years and is far removed from
>   traffic areas.)

Pass all of the ingredients through a juicer. Drink immediately.

Pain-Away Piña Colada

2-inch-thick slice fresh pineapple, core and outer skin removed, chopped into large chunks

One 13.5-ounce can coconut milk (this is one of the only canned foods that is part of the Healing Food Pyramid)

Blend in a blender with 8 to 10 ice cubes. Serve immediately.

Cranberry Antipain Cocktail

This juice, when drunk regularly, helps eliminate inflammation because of the high amount of vitamin C found in the cranberries.

3 apples, chopped into large chunks

1 cup cranberries

Pass all of the ingredients through a juicer. Dilute with water.

Note: If you are using frozen cranberries, juice only the apples, add pure water, and then blend the juice together with the cranberries in a blender. Drink immediately.

Happy Joint Juice

1 cucumber, chopped into large chunks

4 stalks celery

1 to 2 apples, depending on preferred sweetness, chopped into large chunks

Pass all of the ingredients through a juicer. Drink immediately.

Cran-Berry Melon Power Juice

2 large slices of watermelon, chopped into large chunks

½ cup blueberries

½ cup cranberries

Pass all of the ingredients through a juicer. Serve over ice if desired.

Celery-Apple Anti-Inflammatory Juice

4 stalks celery, chopped into large chunks
1 apple, chopped into large chunks

Pass all of the ingredients through a juicer. Serve over ice if desired.

Tropical Enzyme Blast Smoothie

½ papaya, seeded and peeled, chopped into large chunks
1 mango, pitted and peeled, chopped into large chunks
1 frozen banana, chopped into large chunks
1-inch slice fresh pineapple, cored and outer skin removed, chopped into large chunks
1 to 2 cups water, depending on desired consistency

Blend all of the ingredients in a blender or food processor. Serve.

Blue Raspberry Anti-Inflammatory Smoothie

1 cup raspberries, fresh or frozen
1 cup blueberries, fresh or frozen
1 banana, frozen, chopped into large chunks
1½ to 2 cups pure water, depending on desired consistency

Blend all of the ingredients together, and serve.

Almond Milk

¼ cup raw, unsalted almonds
1 cup water
½ teaspoon unpasteurized honey or 2 drops liquid stevia (found in most health food stores)

Blend all of the ingredients together until smooth. Strain through a cheesecloth-lined sieve or an almond milk–making bag (available in many health food stores or online). Drink on its own or use as a base for smoothies.

Pain-Elimination Tea

Purchase dried herbs at your local health food store. Mix together as follows:

¾ cup white willow bark
½ cup juniper berries
¾ cup elder
½ cup primrose flowers

Mix all dried ingredients in a jar for future use. Shake to blend together well. Use 1 teaspoon of the dried herbs in a tea strainer; infuse for 3 to 5 minutes. Drink 3 cups per day. The jar of bulk herbs should last at least 2 to 3 months.

Dr. Cook's Ginger Pain-Relief Tea

This simple and delicious tea can be made in advance and stored in the fridge for about four days. But don't let its simplicity fool you—it has powerful therapeutic effects.

3-inch piece fresh ginger, chopped into small slices
6 cups pure water
Stevia (drops or powder)

Add the ginger to a medium pot of water with the pure water. Bring to a boil, and then reduce the heat to medium-low. Let simmer for at least 30 minutes. Add stevia to taste. I find that 2 drops of stevia per cup of ginger tea is perfect. Drink 3 cups of tea daily for best results.

Antipain Remedy

½ cup organic turmeric (spice available from most health food stores)

½ cup of raw, unpasteurized honey.

Mix turmeric with honey, and store in a sealed jar. Consume 1 teaspoon daily. Alternatively, pour 1 cup of boiled water over 1 teaspoon of the turmeric-honey mixture, and drink as a tea.

HOW TO MAKE AMAZING SALADS

Make salads the focal point of your meals. That might sound boring, but there really are a tremendous number of delectable salads you can make if you vary the ingredients. Here is a list to help you get started. Use your creativity.

mixed greens (mesclun)	grapefruit slices
Romaine lettuce	avocado
Boston lettuce	green peppers
leaf lettuce	red peppers
radicchio	yellow peppers
pea shoots	finely chopped broccoli
alfalfa sprouts	cucumber
broccoli sprouts	olives
onion sprouts	edible flowers
clover sprouts	grated carrots
mung bean sprouts	fresh peas
chickpeas	grated cabbage
kidney beans	chopped parsley
pinto beans	chopped cilantro
lima beans	mushrooms (raw or
Great Northern beans	cooked)
any other type of legume	green onion
sliced strawberries	raspberries
apple slices	blueberries
orange slices	celery

SALADS, SALAD DRESSINGS, AND DIPS

Super-Strengthening Salad Dressing/Dip

This dressing can be used in place of Caesar salad dressing or as a delicious dip for crudités. It is packed with a huge amount of calcium.

½ cup raw tahini (mashed sesame seeds, found in most health food stores or Lebanese or Middle Eastern markets)
2 lemons*
1 fresh garlic clove
1 to 2 tablespoons cold-pressed flax oil
pure water (as needed to obtain the desired consistency)

Blend all of the ingredients together, adding the water until you obtain the desired consistency. Use more water for a salad dressing, less for a vegetable dip.

Note: Do *not* substitute ReaLemon or other lemon products for the lemon juice. These products have been cooked, making them acidic in the body. Fresh lemon is alkalizing to the body, which is essential so as to allow your body to absorb the large amount of calcium in this dressing.

Joint-Healing Guacamole

This recipe makes an excellent veggie dip or sandwich spread. Use soon after making it, or it will discolor.

1 avocado, pitted and peeled
1 small garlic clove
½ lime
Dash Celtic sea salt
1 tablespoon cold-pressed flaxseed oil

Blend all of the ingredients together until creamy, using a hand mixer or food processor. Serve with vegetable crudités, such as carrot, celery, red or green pepper sticks, broccoli, or cauliflower.

Healing Five-Bean Salad

One 15-ounce can cooked mixed beans (such as kidney,
    garbanzo, pinto, etc.), rinsed
2 stalks celery, finely chopped
1 purple onion, finely chopped
1 green pepper, finely chopped
1 red pepper, finely chopped
1 green onion, finely chopped
Handful raw green or yellow beans, chopped
¾ cup cold-pressed flax seed oil (make sure it is refrigerated)
⅓ cup apple cider vinegar (with sediment in the bottom;
    purchase at a health food store)
½ teaspoon Celtic sea salt
1 tablespoon pure maple syrup
½ teaspoon basil
½ teaspoon thyme
½ teaspoon oregano
Dash of cayenne pepper

1. Mix the beans and all of the vegetables together in a
   bowl.
2. In a jar whisk together the remaining ingredients. Pour
   half of the dressing over the bean mixture.
3. For best taste, let marinate overnight or a couple of
   hours. Store the remaining dressing in a sealed jar in the
   refrigerator for later use.

Mexican Salad

1 head leaf or Romaine lettuce, washed and dried
1 tomato, chopped
1 avocado, chopped
Dash Celtic sea salt
Handful fresh cilantro
1 tablespoon cold-pressed flaxseed oil
1 lime
1 small garlic clove

1. Cut or tear the lettuce and place into bowls to form a base for the other salad ingredients.
2. Place the tomato, avocado, salt, cilantro, and oil together in a separate bowl. Squeeze the juice of the lime over the ingredients, and chop or press the garlic into the bowl, and toss together well.
3. Serve the tomato mixture over the salad greens.

Anti-Arthritis Powerhouse Salad Dressing

We need plenty of essential fatty acids for healing. Most people eat harmful fats, and those who eat healthy ones often eat them in an inappropriate ratio. We need both omega 3 and omega 6 fatty acids for health, but most people eat twenty times the amount of omega 6 fatty acids than omega 3s. The problem with this disparity is that, although your body requires omega 6s, too much worsens pain and inflammation. Omega 3s help keep omega 6s in check. This salad dressing is very high in omega 3 fatty acids.

In addition, one of the best foods for arthritic types of pains is apple cider vinegar. I've used this here to maximize the dressing's pain-fighting properties. Be sure to use apple cider vinegar that contains live culture, known as the "mother."

Blueberries are excellent pain fighters as well. They contain a substance that is ten times more potent than aspirin.

½ cup blueberries, fresh or frozen
¾ cup cold-pressed flaxseed oil (make sure it is refrigerated)
⅓ cup apple cider vinegar (with sediment in the bottom;
      purchase at a health food store)
Dash Celtic sea salt
1 tablespoon pure maple syrup

Blend all of the ingredients with a hand mixer or whisk together. If whisking ingredients together, mash the blueberries with a fork.

Note: Pour over mixed baby greens because they have the greatest healing properties of various types of lettuce.

Inflammation-Beating Salad Dressing

¾ cup cold-pressed flaxseed oil (make sure it is
      refrigerated)
⅓ cup apple cider vinegar (with sediment in the bottom;
      purchase at a health food store)
½ teaspoon Celtic sea salt
½ teaspoon basil
½ teaspoon thyme
½ teaspoon oregano
Dash of cayenne pepper

Blend all of the ingredients with a hand mixer or whisk together.

Note: Pour over mixed baby greens because they have the greatest healing properties of various types of lettuce.

COMPLEMENTARY DISHES

Cooked Millet

> 1 cup whole millet
> 2½ cups pure water
> Dash olive oil
> Dash Celtic sea salt

Place all of the ingredients into a pot; cover and bring to a boil. Reduce heat to low, and let simmer for 45 minutes. Serve on its own or as a base for steamed or stir-fried vegetables.

Mexican Bruschetta

> 1 tomato, chopped
> 1 avocado, chopped
> 1 small garlic clove, pressed or finely chopped
> Dash Celtic sea salt
> Handful fresh cilantro
> 1 tablespoon cold-pressed flaxseed oil (make sure it is
>   refrigerated)
> ½ lime
> 4 slices 100 percent whole-grain gluten-free bread,
>   toasted

Mix all of the other ingredients through the oil into a bowl. Squeeze the lime juice over the ingredients, and then toss together. Spoon the tomato mixture over the toast, and serve.

Veggie Wrap

Joint-Healing Guacamole (page 185)
2 to 4 soft tortilla shells (preservative- and gluten-free)
1 to 2 carrots, shredded
½ cucumber, sliced
½ red and/or green bell pepper, sliced into strips
1 to 2 tomatoes, sliced

Spread the guacamole into the center of the tortilla shells. Place a handful of each raw vegetable in a line in the center of the tortilla, roll into a wrap, and enjoy.

Note: If you don't want to use tomatoes or bell peppers, substitute your favorite raw vegetables, sliced, chopped, or grated.

Ultimate Joint-Healing Curry (Lentil Dahl)

This is a delicious lentil curry dish. I modified the traditional recipe slightly to give it even greater injury-healing properties. Even if you're not a huge fan of lentils, give this healing recipe a try.

1 yam, cubed
2 tablespoons extra-virgin olive oil
1 large onion, chopped
½ teaspoon mustard seeds
4 dried red chilies
1-inch piece ginger, grated
2 garlic cloves, chopped
3 cups cooked lentils (or two 15-ounce cans, rinsed)
½ teaspoon turmeric
1 teaspoon Celtic sea salt
Fresh cilantro, if desired

1. Boil the cubed yams in water in a medium to large pot until they are soft. Pour off the excess water, leaving

enough to mash the yams with a hand blender until it has a smooth consistency.

2. Heat the olive oil over low heat in a frying pan, then cook the onion, mustard seeds, chilies, ginger, and garlic until the onion becomes transparent.

3. Add the onion mixture to the yams, then add the lentils, turmeric, salt and ½ cup water; stir together. Let simmer over low heat until it is warmed and the flavors mingle. Serve in bowls with fresh cilantro as a garnish.

DESSERTS

Cashew Cream

    1 cup raw, unsalted cashews
    ½ to 1 cup pure water, depending on desired consistency of cream
    2 teaspoons unpasteurized honey

Blend all of the ingredients together until creamy. Serve with fresh blueberries, strawberries, or other fruit.

Berry Blast Ice Cream

    1 cup raspberries, frozen
    1 cup blueberries, frozen
    2 bananas, frozen

Blend all of the ingredients in a food processor or push through a Champion juicer with the blank screen.

Also by Michelle Schoffro Cook, PhD, DNM, ROHP

Print Books

Be Your Own Herbalist: Essential Herbs for Health, Beauty, and Cooking (New World Library)

Boost Your Brain Power in 60 Seconds: The 4-Week Plan for a Sharper Mind, Better Memory, and Healthier Brain (Rodale)

The 4-Week Ultimate Body Detox Plan: A Program for Greater Energy, Health, and Vitality (Wiley)

The Probiotic Promise: Simple Steps to Heal Your Body from the Inside Out (DaCapo)

60 Seconds to Slim: Balance Your Body Chemistry to Burn Fat Fast (Rodale)

The Ultimate pH Solution: Balance Your Body Chemistry to Prevent Disease and Lose Weight (HarperCollins)

Weekend Wonder Detox: Quick Cleanses to Strengthen Your Body and Enhance Your Beauty (DaCapo)

E-books

Acid-Alkaline Food Chart

Cancer-Proof: All-Natural Solutions for Cancer Prevention and Healing

Everything You Need to Know About Healthy Eating

Healing Recipes

The Vitality Diet: 21 Days to a Leaner, Healthier, Happier, More Energetic You

Notes

CHAPTER 1

1 Joseph Mercola, DO, "Death from Prescription Drugs: The New Epidemic Sweeping Across America," October 26, 2011, http://articles.mercola.com/sites/articles/archive/2011/10/26/prescription-drugs-number-one-cause-preventable-death-in-us.aspx.

2 Verispan, "Vital Signs: Top 10 Drugs Prescribed by Rheumatologists," *Rheumatology News*, www.rheumatologynews.com/article/S1541-9800%2808%2970348-X/pdf.

3 "Methotrexate Side-Effects," Drugs.com, www.drugs.com/sfx/methotrexate-side-effects.html.

4 Alan R. Gaby, MD, and the Healthnotes Medical Team, *A-Z Guide to Drug-Herb-Vitamin Interactions: Revised and Expanded 2nd Edition: Improve Your Health and Avoid Side Effects When Using Common Medications and Natural Supplements Together* (New York: Three Rivers Press, 2008), 170.

5 Ibid., 170.

6 "Prednisone Side-Effects," Drugs.com, www.drugs.com/sfx/prednisone-side-effects.html.

7 Gaby, *A-Z Guide to Drug-Herb-Vitamin Interactions*, 200.

8 Ibid.

9 Ibid., 201.

10 "Hydroxychloroquine Side-Effects," Drugs.com, www.drugs
   .com/sfx/hydroxychloroquine-side-effects.html.

11 Gaby, *A-Z Guide to Drug-Herb-Vitamin Interactions*, 201.

12 "Hydrocodone Side-Effects," Drugs.com, www.drugs.com/
   sfx/hydrocodone-side-effects.html, accessed January 5, 2016.

13 "Acetaminophen Side-Effects," Drugs.com, www.drugs.com/
   sfx/acetaminophen-side-effects.html.

14 Gaby, *A-Z Guide to Drug-Herb-Vitamin Interactions*, 4.

15 Ibid.

16 "Tramadol Side-Effects," Drugs.com, www.drugs.com/sfx/
   tramadol-side-effects.html.

17 Gaby, *A-Z Guide to Drug-Herb-Vitamin Interactions*, 266–7.

18 Jeffrey S. Bland, *The Disease Delusion: Conquering the Causes
   of Chronic Illness for a Healthier, Longer, and Happier Life*
   (New York: Harper Collins), 39–40.

19 Bahar Gholipour, "Placebo Effect May Account for Half of
   Drug's Efficacy," *LiveScience*, January 8, 2014, www.livescience
   .com/42430-placebo-effect-half-of-drug-efficacy.html.

20 Bill Sardi, "Does Anybody Still Believe Slam Pieces on Dietary
   Supplements?" *Orthomolecular Medicine News Service*,
   August 13, 2012. http://www.orthomolecular.org/resources/
   omns/v08n27.shtml, accessed February 29, 2016.

21 Bland. *The Disease Delusion*, 69.

CHAPTER 2

1 "Chapter 2: Profiling Food Consumption in America," *Agriculture Fact Book*, US Department of Agriculture, www.usda
   .gov/factbook/chapter2.pdf.

2 Leslie Ridgeway, "High Fructose Corn Syrup Linked to Diabetes," *USC News*, https://news.usc.edu/44415/high-fructose
   -corn-syrup-linked-to-diabetes.

3   Mark Hyman, "5 Reasons High Fructose Corn Syrup Will
    Kill You," http://drhyman.com/blog/2011/05/13/5-reasons-high
    -fructose-corn-syrup-will-kill-you.

4   Ibid.

5   Ibid.

6   Leslie Ridgeway, "High Fructose Corn Syrup Linked to Dia-
    betes," *USC News*, November 28, 2012, https://news.usc.edu/
    44415/high-fructose-corn-syrup-linked-to-diabetes.

7   Ibid.

8   D. I. Jalal, G. Smits, R. J. Johnson, and M. Chonchol, "Increased
    Fructose Associates with Elevated Blood Pressure," *Journal
    of the American Society of Nephrology* 21, no. 9 (September
    2010): 1543–9.

9   Jonathan Suez, Tal Korem, David Zeevi, Gili Zilberman-
    Schapira, Christoph A. Thaiss, Ori Maza, David Isreali et al.,
    "Artificial Sweeteners Induce Glucose Intolerance by Alter-
    ing Gut Microbiota," *Nature* 514, no. 7521 (October 9, 2014):
    181–6.

10 Robert O. Young and Shelley Redford Young, *The pH Miracle:
    Balance Your Diet, Reclaim Your Health* (New York: Warner
    Books, 2002).

11 J. A. Levy, A. B. Ibrahim, T. Shirai, K. Ohta, R. Gagasawa, H.
    Yoshida, J. Estes, and M. Gardner, "Dietary Fat Affects Immune
    Response, Production of Antiviral Factors, and Immune Com-
    plex Disease in NZP/NZW Mice," *Proceedings of the National
    Academy of Sciences* 79, no. 6 (March 1982): 1974–8.

12 J. Kjeldsen-Kragh, M. Haugen, C. F. Borchgrevink, E. Laerum,
    M. Eek, P. Mowinkel, K. Hovi, and O. Förre "Controlled Trial
    of Fasting and One Year Vegetarian Diet in Rheumatoid
    Arthritis," *Lancet* 338, no. 8772 (October 1991): 899–902.

13 S. Ahmed, N. Wang, B. B. Hafeez, V. K. Cherunu, and T. M.
    Haggi, "Punica granatum L. Extract Inhibits IL-1Beta-
    Induced Expression of Matrix Metalloproteinases by Inhib-
    iting the Activation of MAP Kinases and NF-kB in Human

Chondrocytes In Vitro," *Journal of Nutrition* 135, no. 9 (September 2005): 2096–102.

14 O. A. Fawole, N. P. Makunga, and U. L. Opara, "Antibacterial, Antioxidant, and Tyrosinase-Inhibition Activities of Pomegranate Fruit Peel Methanolic Extract," *BMC Complementary and Alternative Medicine* (October 2012); Irene Alexandraki and Carlos Palacio, "Gram Negative versus Gram Positive Bacteremia: What Is More Alarming?" *Critical Care* 14, no. 3 (May 2010): 1–2.

CHAPTER 3

1 Canadian Society for Orthomolecular Medicine (CSOM), "Canadian Society for Orthomolecular Medicine," www .csom.ca.

2 Linus Pauling, "Orthomolecular Psychiatry: Varying the Concentrations of Substances Normally Present in the Human Body May Control Mental Disease," *Science* 160, no. 3825 (April 19, 1968): 265–71.

3 "Vitamin," Oxford Dictionaries, www.oxforddictionaries.com/ definition/english/vitamin.

4 "Niacin and Niacinamide (Vitamin B3)," MedlinePlus, www .nlm.nih.gov/medlineplus/druginfo/natural/924.html.

5 James South, "SAMe—The Ultimate Nutrient for Mood, Liver, Heart, Joint, and Brain Protection," www.antiaging-systems .com/articles/221-same-the-ultimate-nutrient-for-mood-liver -heart-joint-and-brain-protection.

6 Patrick Holford, *The New Optimum Nutrition Bible* (London: Crossing Press, 2004), 142–3.

7 Ibid., 137, 139.

8 Elson M. Haas and Buck Levin, *Staying Healthy with Nutrition: The Complete Guide to Diet and Nutritional Medicine* (Berkeley, CA: Celestial Arts, 2006), 655.

9 Holford, *The New Optimum Nutrition Bible*, 138.

10 A. Yxfeldt, S. Wållberg-Jonsson, J. Hultdin, and S. Rantapää-Dahlqvist, "Homocysteine in Patients with Rheumatoid Arthritis in Relation to Inflammation and B-Vitamin Treatment," *Scandinavian Journal of Rheumatology* 32, no. 4 (2003): 205–10.

11 Haas and Levin, *Staying Healthy with Nutrition*, 655.

12 K. R. Gough, C. McCarthy, A. E. Read, D. L. Mollin, and A. H. Waters, "Folic Acid Deficiency in Rheumatoid Arthritis," *British Medical Journal* 1, no. 5377 (January 1964): 212–7.

13 "Folate," Arthritis Foundation, www.arthritis.org/living-with-arthritis/treatments/natural/vitamins-minerals/guide/folate.php.

14 "Vitamin B12," Arthritis Foundation, www.arthritis.org/living-with-arthritis/treatments/natural/vitamins-minerals/guide/vitamin-b-12.php.

CHAPTER 4

1 Brian R. Clement. *Living Foods for Optimum Health: Staying Healthy in an Unhealthy World* (Roseville, CA: Prima Health, 1998), 39.

2 Anthony J. Cichoke, *Enzymes and Enzyme Therapy: How to Jump Start Your Way to Lifelong Good Health* (Los Angeles, CA: Keats Publishing, 2000), 163.

3 C. Steffen, J. Smolen, I. Hörger, and J. Menzel, "Enzymtherapie im vergleich mit immunkomplexbestimmungen bei chronischer polyarthritis." *Zeitschr. f. Rheumatologie* 44 (1985): 51–6.

4 P. Streichhan et al., "Resorption partikulärer und makromolekularer Darminhaltsstoffe." *Nature- und Ganzheitsmedizin* 1 (1988): 90.

5 A. H. M. Viswanatha Swamy and P. A. Patil. "Effect of Some Clinically-Used Proteolytic Enzymes on Inflammation in Rats" *Indian Journal of Pharmaceutical Sciences*, January-February 2008,

http://www.ncbi.nlm.nih.gov/pmc/articles/PMC2852049/, accessed February 29, 2016.

CHAPTER 5

1 Phyllis A. Balch and James F. Balch, *Prescription for Nutritional Healing*, 3rd ed. (New York: Avery, 2000), 72.

2 Bob Capelli and Gerald R. Cysewski, *Astaxanthin: Natural Astaxanthin: King of the Carotenoids* (Kailua-Kona, HI: Cyanotech Corporation, 2007), 19.

3 Ibid., 31–2.

4 Ibid., 35.

5 N. Mncwangi, W. Chen, I. Vermaak, A. M. Viljoen, and N. Gericke, "Devil's Claw—A Review of the Ethnobotany, Phytochemistry, and Biological Activity of *Harpagophytum procumbens*," *Journal of Ethnopharmacology* 143, no. 3 (October 11, 2012): 755–71.

6 "Devil's Claw," WebMD, www.webmd.com/vitamins -supplements/ingredientmono-984-DEVIL'S%20CLAW.aspx ?activeIngredientId=984&activeIngredientName=DEVIL %27S%20CLAW.

7 R. D. Altman and K. C. Marcussen, "Effects of a Ginger Extract on Knee Pain in Patients with Osteoarthritis," *Arthritis and Rheumatism* 44, no. 11 (November 2001): 2531–8.

8 V. N. Drozdov, V. A. Kim, E. V. Tkachenko, and G. G. Varvanina, "Influence of a Specific Ginger Combination on Gastropathy Conditions in Patients with Osteoarthritis of the Knee or Hip," *Journal of Alternative and Complementary Medicine* 18, no. 8 (June 2012): 583–8.

9 S. Ribel-Madsen, E. M. Bartels, A. Stockmarr, A. Borgwards, C. Cornett, B. Danneskiold-Samsøe, and H. Bliddal, "A Synoviocyte Model for Osteoarthritis and Rheumatoid Arthritis: Response to Ibuprofen, Betamethasone, and Ginger

Extract—A Cross-Sectional In Vitro Study," *Arthritis* 2012, no. 5 (2013): 1–9.

10 K. C. Srivastava and T. Mustafa, "Ginger (Zingiber officinalis) in Rheumatism and Musculoskeletal Disorders," *Medical Hypotheses* 39, no. 4 (December 1992): 342–8.

11 Ibid.

12 Ibid.

13 Y. Takada, A. Bhardwaj, P. Potdar, and B. B. Aggarwal, "Nonsteroidal Anti-Inflammatory Agents Differ in Their Ability to Suppress NF-kappaB Activation, Inhibition of Expression of Cyclooxygenase-2 and Cyclin D1and Abrogation of Tumor Cell Proliferation," *Oncogene* 23, no. 57 (December 2004): 9247–58.

14 F. Di Pierro et al. "Comparative Evaluation of the Pain-Relieving Properties of a Lecithinized Formulation of Curcumin (Meriva®), Nimesulide, and Acetaminophen," *Journal of Pain Research* 6 (2013): 201–5.

15   F. Di Pierro et al. "Comparative Evaluation of the Pain-Relieving Properties of a Lecithinized Formulation of Curcumin (Meriva®), Nimesulide, and Acetaminophen," *Journal of Pain Research* 6 (2013): 201–5.

16 Joseph N. Sciberras et al. "The Effect of Turmeric (Curcumin) Supplementation on Cytokine and Inflammatory Marker Responses Following 2 hours of Endurance Cycling." *Journal of the International Society of Sports Nutrition*, August 12, 2014. http://jissn.biomedcentral.com/articles/10.1186/s12970 –014–0066–3, accessed February 29, 2016.

17 F. Drobnic, J. Riera, G. Appendino, S. Togni, F. Francheschi. X. Valle, A. Pons et al., "Reduction of Delayed Onset Muscle Soreness by a Novel Curcumin Delivery System (Meriva): A Randomised, Placebo-Controlled Trial," *Journal of the International Society of Sports Nutrition* 11 (June 2014): 31.

18 Ananya Mandal, "What Are Cytokines?" NewsMedical, May 17, 2014, www.news-medical.net/health/What-are -Cytokines.aspx.

19 Alan C. Logan, *The Brain Diet: The Connections Between Nutrition, Mental Health, and Intelligence* (Nashville, TN: Cumberland House Publishing, 2006), 114.

20 David M. Marquis, "Inflammation Affects Every Aspect of Your Health," Mercola, March 7, 2013, http://articles.mercola.com/sites/articles/archive/2013/03/07/inflammation-triggers-disease-symptoms.aspx.

21 Ibid.

22 Ibid.

23 Jacob Teitelbaum, *From Fatigued to Fantastic!* (New York: Avery, 2007).

24 Cobi Slater, *The Ultimate Candida Guide and Cookbook: The Breakthrough Plan for Eliminating Disease-Causing Yeast and Revolutionizing Your Health: Including Over 150 Candida Fighting Recipes* (Maitland, FL: Xulon Press, 2014), 11.

25 Michelle Schoffro Cook, *The Probiotic Promise: Simple Steps to Heal Your Body from the Inside Out* (Boston, MA: DaCapo, 2015).

26 Slater, *The Ultimate Candida Guide and Cookbook*, 16.

27 Michelle Schoffro Cook, *60 Seconds to Slim: Balance Your Body Chemistry to Burn Fat Fast!* (Emmaus, PA: Rodale, 2013), 184–8; Slater, *The Ultimate Candida Guide and Cookbook*, 16.

28 Nina Lincoff, "Gut Bacteria May Cause Inflammation in Rheumatoid Arthritis," HealthlineNews, November 8, 2013, www.healthline.com/health-news/arthritis-gut-bacteria-may-trigger-ra-110813.

29 Ibid.

30 L. Pineda Mde, S. F. Thompson, K. Summers, F. de Leon, J. Pope, and G. Reid, "A Randomized, Double-Blind, Placebo-Controlled Pilot Study of Probiotics in Active Rheumatoid Arthritis," *Medical Science Monitor* 17, no. 6 (June 2011): CR347–54.

31 Klaire Labs, "The Probiotic Leader: Functions of Probiotic Species," www.klaire.com/probioticleader3.htm.

32 Ibid.

33 H. J. Kang and S. H. Im, "Probiotics as an Immune Modulator," *Journal of Nutritional Science and Vitaminology* (Tokyo) 61 Suppl. (2015): S103–5.

CHAPTER 7

1 Christiane Staiger, "Comfrey: A Clinical Overview," *Phytotherapy Research* 26, no. 10 (October 2012); 1441–8.

CHAPTER 8

1 "'Dirty Dozen' Cosmetic Chemicals to Avoid," David Suzuki Foundation, www.davidsuzuki.org/issues/health/science/toxics/dirty-dozen-cosmetic-chemicals/?gclid=CKPI2rPgvsECFQcSMwodfG4A3Q.

2 Tracey Lapetina, "Estrogen Dominance and Joint Pain," eHow. www.ehow.com/facts_5475511_estrogen-dominance-joint-pain.html.

3 "'Dirty Dozen' Cosmetic Chemicals to Avoid."

4 "'Dirty Dozen' Cosmetic Chemicals to Avoid."

5 "Parabens," David Suzuki Foundation, http://davidsuzuki.org/issues/health/science/toxics/chemicals-in-your-cosmetics-parabens.

6 "'Dirty Dozen' Cosmetic Chemicals to Avoid."

7 J. Lee et al. "Sedentary Behavior and Physical Function: Objective Evidence from the Osteoarthritis Initiative," *Arthritis Care and Research* (Hoboken) 67, no. 3 (March 2015): 366–73.

Resources

OTHER RECOMMENDED READING

Michael Castleman. *The New Healing Herbs: The Classic Guide to Nature's Best Medicines Featuring the Top 100 Time-Tested Herbs*. New York: Bantam Books, 2002.

James A. Duke. *The Green Pharmacy: The Ultimate Compendium of Natural Remedies from the World's Foremost Authority on Healing Herbs*. New York: Rodale, 1997.

David Hoffman. *Medical Herbalism: The Science and Practice of Herbal Medicine*. Rochester, VT: Healing Arts Press, 2003.

Terry Willard, *Edible and Medicinal Plants of the Rocky Mountains and Neighbouring Territories*. Calgary: Wild Rose College of Natural Medicine, 1992.

AROMATHERAPY AND HERBAL SUPPLIES

There are some excellent companies that offer dried or bulk herbs for use in your aromatherapy oils and creams or herbs for teas. Two of my favorite suppliers follow.

Harmonic Arts offers a wide range of herbs and natural foods and some amazing medicinal herb blends. Yarrow and

Angela Willard, the founders of Harmonic Arts, also offer many instructional and entertaining videos worth checking out on their website, https://harmonicarts.ca/ref/65.

Mountain Rose Herbs offers a range of herbs and aroma-therapy products worth checking out. Visit them at www .mountainroseherbs.com/index.php?AID=13769.

Index

About the Author

Michelle Schoffro Cook, PhD, DNM, DHS, ROHP, is the author of nineteen health books, including the international best-sellers *60 Seconds to Slim, The Ultimate pH Solution,* and *The 4-Week Ultimate Body Detox Plan.* Her books have been translated into many languages, including Spanish, Greek, Chinese, Thai, Indonesian, and Russian. She holds advanced degrees in natural health, holistic and orthomolecular nutrition, and traditional natural medicine and has twenty-five years of experience in the field. Dr. Cook is a board-certified doctor of natural medicine who has received the Doctor of Humanitarian Services designation from the World Organization of Natural Medicine and a World-Leading Intellectual Award for her contribution to natural medicine. She is a regular blogger for CulturedCook.com and Care2.com. Visit her websites DrMichelleCook.com and WorldsHealthiestDiet.com.

World's Healthiest News

You can subscribe to Dr. Schoffro Cook's free e-zine, *World's Healthiest News,* to obtain natural health insights, news, research, recipes, and more. Each edition features natural approaches to boost your energy, supercharge your immune system, and look and feel great. Subscribe at WorldsHealthiestDiet.com.

Dr. Cook's Blogs

Don't miss a single blog by Dr. Cook; follow her at:

DrMichelleCook.com
CulturedCook.com
HealthySurvivalist.com
Care2.com/GreenLiving/author/MCook

E-Books

Discover Dr. Cook's exclusive e-books on her site, Worlds
HealthiestDiet.com
Follow her on:

Twitter @mschoffrocook
Facebook facebook.com/drschoffrocook
Pinterest pinterest.com/drmichellecook